ESSENTIALS

# PROMOTING HEALTH AND WELLBEING

For Nursing and Healthcare Students

**Note to readers:** throughout the book, and especially in many of the *Activities*, you will notice the use of quicklinks, such as bit.ly/2-9A

We have used these shortened versions to save you having to re-key long web addresses. Just type them into any browser and you will be taken straight to the relevant webpage. In the case of the sample quicklink above, this will take you to the NHS *Why 5 a day?* healthy eating advice at www.nhs.uk/live-well/eat-well/why-5-a-day/?tabname=food-and-diet

ESSENTIALS

# PROMOTING HEALTH AND WELLBEING

For Nursing and Healthcare Students

Edited by
**CLARE BENNETT**
and
**SUE LILLYMAN**

Lantern

ISBN: 9781908625854

Lantern Publishing Ltd, The Old Hayloft, Vantage Business Park, Bloxham Rd, Banbury, OX16 9UX, UK
www.lanternpublishing.com

© 2020, Clare Bennett, Sue Lillyman, Judith Carrier, Sarah Fry, Lucy Hope, Alison H. James, Beverley Johnson, Anneyce Knight, Michelle Moseley, Nita Muir, Stephen Scott, Gemma Stacey-Emile, Lisa Stephens and Katharine Whittingham

The right of Clare Bennett, Sue Lillyman, Judith Carrier, Sarah Fry, Lucy Hope, Alison H. James, Beverley Johnson, Anneyce Knight, Michelle Moseley, Nita Muir, Stephen Scott, Gemma Stacey-Emile, Lisa Stephens and Katharine Whittingham to be identified as authors of this work has been asserted by them in accordance with the Copyright, Design and Patents Act 1988.

**British Library Cataloguing in Publication Data**
A catalogue record for this book is available from the British Library

The authors and publisher have made every attempt to ensure the content of this book is up to date and accurate. However, healthcare knowledge and information is changing all the time so the reader is advised to double-check any information in this text on drug usage, treatment procedures, the use of equipment, etc. to confirm that it complies with the latest safety recommendations, standards of practice and legislation, as well as local Trust policies and procedures. Students are advised to check with their tutor and/or practice supervisor before carrying out any of the procedures in this textbook.

Cover design by Andrew Magee Design Ltd
Typeset by Andrew Magee Design Ltd
Printed in the UK
Last digit is the print number: 10 9 8 7 6 5 4 3

# Contents

About the authors . . . . . . vii

Abbreviations . . . . . . xi

Introduction . . . . . . xiii

1 Theoretical perspectives: health promotion, health education and public health . . . . . . 1

2 Behaviour change: theories, models and approaches . . . . . . 21

3 Inequalities in health . . . . . . 45

4 Global health and wellbeing . . . . . . 69

5 Enabling, mediating and advocating in health promotion . . . . . . 85

6 Building a healthy public policy . . . . . . 103

7 Advocating mental health promotion . . . . . . 121

8 Strengthening community action . . . . . . 139

9 Professional responsibilities of the nurse as a health promoter . . . . . . 153

10 Leadership for health promotion . . . . . . 167

11 Evidence-based health promotion . . . . . . 183

Index . . . . . . 197

# About the authors

**Clare Bennett** is a registered nurse with a background in immunology, HIV, infectious diseases and sexual health. She is currently a senior lecturer at Cardiff University and teaches health promotion, public health, leadership and quality improvement on undergraduate and postgraduate programmes for nurses and allied health professionals. Clare is also an honorary lecturer at the University of Freiburg, Germany. She is an active researcher in the field of sexual health promotion, teaches research methods and supervises doctoral students. She is widely published in academic journals and has co-authored three textbooks.

**Sue Lillyman** is a registered nurse and midwife with a background in older people, end of life, long-term conditions and care of people with dementia and frailty. She is currently working as an associate lecturer for the University of Worcester and as programme lead for Education for Health. Sue also teaches management and leadership in healthcare, teaching and learning for clinical practice, reflective practice and ethical issues. She is an active researcher in the fields of international students, student exchange and end of life issues. She is widely published in academic books and journals.

**Judith Carrier** is a reader in primary care/public health nursing and director of the Wales Centre for Evidence Based Care – a JBI Centre of Excellence, at Cardiff University School of Healthcare Sciences. Research and teaching interests include evidence synthesis and utilisation and long-term condition management. Judith has published several systematic reviews in addition to a textbook on the management of long-term conditions in primary care. Her PhD focused on the social organisation of practice nurses' use of knowledge. Her clinical background was in practice nursing, where she specialised in the care of people with diabetes. Judith has presented at several national and international conferences on systematic review methods and long-term conditions and is a senior associate editor for the *JBI Evidence Synthesis* journal.

**Sarah Fry** is a lecturer and nurse with expertise in minority ethnic health and community engagement. Sarah worked in emergency medicine before working as a prostate cancer research nurse, which is where her interest in minority ethnic health developed. Sarah started a PhD in 2013 focusing on oncology, men's health and community-developed perceptions of prostate cancer risk. The PhD was awarded in

2017 and Sarah carried out extensive community engagement work during her PhD, which has led to expertise relating to community-driven health action.

**Lucy Hope** is a registered midwife and senior lecturer in midwifery in the College of Health, Life and Environmental Sciences at the University of Worcester. She has experience in teaching across the undergraduate midwifery degree programme and is a PhD supervisor. Lucy has worked in a variety of clinical midwifery settings and gained considerable experience working as a midwifery researcher at the University of Birmingham on projects evaluating the effectiveness of peer support for breastfeeding and the support of pregnant women with identified social risk. Latterly she also worked as a research midwife for the National Institute for Health Research reproductive health and childbirth speciality group. In 2014 Lucy was awarded a PhD which focused on evaluating the effect of peer support for breastfeeding, utilising both quantitative and qualitative methodologies.

**Alison James** is a senior lecturer and doctorate student in the School of Healthcare Sciences at Cardiff University, teaching across the undergraduate and postgraduate programmes in adult nursing and healthcare sciences. She is a Registered General Nurse with a clinical background in neurosciences, critical care and clinical research in Creutzfeldt–Jakob disease and osteoporosis. She began her academic career in 2008 in knowledge transfer and postgraduate teaching in leadership and management in health and social care at the Institute of Public Care, Oxford Brookes University. Her special interests include leadership, action learning and interprofessional learning.

**Beverley Johnson** is an adult nursing lecturer in the School of Healthcare Sciences at Cardiff University and the Professional Head for nursing. She has a BA in adult nursing and an MSc in sociology. Beverley's clinical background is in critical care and she has led a widening access project in the community. Beverley is currently working on quality improvement in Malawi and her teaching interests are sociology and inequalities in health.

**Anneyce Knight**, as a registered nurse, previously worked within the NHS and then moved into higher education in 2000. At the University of Greenwich, as programme leader for the BSc in health and combined studies, she led on the development of the then innovative BSc health and wellbeing. Currently, Anneyce is Acting Associate Dean for Global Engagement at Bournemouth University (Faculty of Health and Social Sciences). As part of her teaching portfolio she lectures on wellbeing, health promotion and public health. Her main research interest relates to wellbeing, presenting and writing papers nationally and internationally, as well as being co-editor of three books.

**Michelle Moseley** is a registered nurse with vast experience in children's nursing, health visiting and as a lead nurse for safeguarding children. Since obtaining her master's degree in 2012 she has worked as a lecturer in primary care and public health nursing within the School of Healthcare Sciences, Cardiff University, where she is also undertaking a PhD applicable to health visiting practice and safeguarding supervision. Michelle's passion is health visiting, working with families with children

0–5 years in promoting health and wellbeing, as well as the safeguarding of children and young people.

**Nita Muir** is a principal lecturer at the University of Brighton; she is a registered nurse, has a doctorate in education and is a senior fellow with AdvanceHE. Her current role is as the academic lead for the pre-registration nursing courses and she teaches a range of contemporary subjects in undergraduate and postgraduate programmes which includes global health, education for health professionals, research and professional knowledge. Nita has worked clinically in a range of acute and community settings both in the UK and internationally; she is a specialist community practitioner and regularly engages with community nurse settings. Her research interests are associated with organisational learning, particularly within the context of nursing. She is interested both in the individual's resilience throughout learning and how wider organisations support this in researching learning *about*, *through* and *at* work.

**Stephen Scott** is a mental health lecturer at Cardiff University. He is a registered nurse in mental health and general nursing and is also accredited as an integrative counsellor and cognitive behavioural therapist. Stephen has led master's level programmes in supervision and reflective practice as well as nursing and primary care mental health training for improving access to psychological therapy practitioners. He joined the team in Cardiff in 2018 and works across the pre-registration nursing programme. His interests span primary care mental health and acute mental health provision and his current practice is focused on cognitive behavioural intervention to promote behavioural change across a wide variety of presentations.

**Gemma Stacey-Emile** is a registered mental health nurse with a background of working within substance misuse services. She is currently a lecturer at Cardiff University and teaches on substance misuse, communication skills, leadership and quality improvement on the undergraduate and postgraduate programmes for nurses and allied health professionals. Gemma has a keen interest in reducing mental health stigma, promoting compassionate care and working at an international level to learn and share experiences and knowledge.

**Lisa Stephens** is a registered nurse and midwife and has occupied various clinical, managerial, teaching and governance positions. In addition, she has held roles in sexual health and teenage pregnancy. She is programme lead on the BSc (Hons) midwifery programme and lead midwife for education at the College of Health, Life and Environmental Sciences at the University of Worcester. She is also a physical activity clinical champion for Public Health England. She has developed and led postgraduate modules on reproductive health and health promotion and is committed to ensuring that student midwives have a full understanding of their role in public health. Lisa has always had a passion for maternal public health, particularly breastfeeding and maternal obesity.

**Katharine Whittingham** is assistant professor at the University of Nottingham and is experienced in leading innovative curriculum development, reflecting her clinical and public health expertise. She previously worked as a health promotion specialist influencing public health policy development, implementing and evaluating projects including the smoking cessation service. Katharine is a member of Public Health England Cardiovascular Disease Prevention Board working to ensure the contribution of nursing is recognised and embedded in policy and service development. She is a member of the Institute of Health Promotion and Education. Katharine has advanced knowledge of research methods in nursing practice as demonstrated through doctoral studies.

# Abbreviations

| | |
|---|---|
| ACE | adverse childhood experiences |
| ACT | acceptance and commitment therapy |
| BAME | black, Asian, minority ethnic |
| CHV | community health volunteer |
| COM | capacity, opportunity and motivation |
| DNA | deoxyribonucleic acid |
| EBHC | evidence-based healthcare |
| EBM | evidence-based medicine |
| EBP | evidence-based practice |
| ED | Emergency Department |
| EI | emotional intelligence |
| FGM | female genital mutilation |
| GP | general practitioner |
| HCP | healthcare practitioner |
| HIA | health impact assessment |
| HIV | human immunodeficiency virus |
| HNA | health needs assessment |
| HPV | human papillomavirus |
| ICN | International Council of Nurses |
| JSNA | joint strategic needs assessment |
| LMIC | low- and middle-income country |
| MDG | Millennium Development Goal |
| MECC | Making Every Contact Count |

*Abbreviations*

| | |
|---|---|
| MMR | measles, mumps and rubella |
| MRSA | methicillin-resistant *Staphylococcus aureus* |
| MSK | musculoskeletal |
| NHS | National Health Service |
| NICE | National Institute for Health and Care Excellence |
| NMC | Nursing and Midwifery Council |
| ONS | Office for National Statistics |
| PHE | Public Health England |
| QOL | quality of life |
| RCN | Royal College of Nursing |
| RN | registered nurse |
| SDG | Sustainable Development Goal |
| SMART | specific, measurable, achievable, realistic and time-bound |
| TB | tuberculosis |
| UN | United Nations |
| WHO | World Health Organization |

# Introduction

Welcome to *Promoting Health and Wellbeing*. This book has been written primarily for student nurses and nursing associates; however, the discussions are equally relevant to student midwives, allied health and social care students. It is also suitable for all health and social care professionals who are new to health promotion.

Health promotion is central to contemporary healthcare practice. This book provides you with an overview of the most relevant theories and policy initiatives. Through the activities that are included in each chapter, you will also learn how to apply these to your daily practice. The book commences with an overview of the theoretical perspectives of health promotion, health education and public health. You are then introduced to behaviour change, inequalities in health, global health and wellbeing and the World Health Organization's strategies for health promotion across the lifespan. The book moves on to examining healthy public policy, promoting mental health and wellbeing, strengthening community action, the professional responsibilities of the nurse in health promotion, leadership for health promotion and evidence-based health promotion.

This book has been designed to enable you to address the outcomes of the NMC's (2018) *Standards of Proficiency for Registered Nurses* second platform 'Promoting health and preventing ill health'. Throughout the book, the discussions are underpinned by relevant psychological, sociological and nursing theory. The book can be read in sequence or as stand-alone chapters. Regardless of how you read it, to get the most out of your reading we encourage you to engage with the activities and case studies in each chapter, as these have been included to help you extend your understanding of how the various concepts relate to nursing practice.

All of the authors who have contributed to this book have a wealth of practice and educational experience and they are passionate about using health promotion theory and policy to enhance the health and wellbeing of individuals and populations. We do hope you enjoy reading this book and that your learning makes a positive contribution to how you carry out health promotion in practice.

Clare Bennett and Sue Lillyman, Editors

# Chapter 1
# Theoretical perspectives: health promotion, health education and public health

Lucy Hope and Lisa Stephens

> **LEARNING OUTCOMES**
>
> When you have finished this chapter, you should be able to:
>
> **1.1** Define the concepts of 'health' and 'wellbeing'
>
> **1.2** Discuss health promotion, health education and public health
>
> **1.3** Describe how the lay concepts of health are relevant for nursing care
>
> **1.4** Outline the fundamental influences on wider determinants of health and wellbeing.

## 1.1 Introduction

The concepts of health promotion, health education and public health are central to nursing practice. In this chapter we introduce these concepts and their foundations in the context of contemporary practice. Social and political drivers that influence decisions and practices surrounding health will be introduced and links to relevant national and international organisations in the field will be explored. Models of health will be presented to help you consider your views on health and wellbeing and examples will be given highlighting a holistic approach to health.

## 1.2 Defining physical and psychological health and wellbeing

The Nursing and Midwifery Council (NMC) (2018a) highlights that registered nurses have a key role in promoting the health and wellbeing of people, families, communities and populations. When exploring the principles of health promotion, health education and public health, it is valuable to first consider what health and wellbeing are in the context of nursing and what the terms incorporate.

> **ACTIVITY 1.1**
>
> Understanding the concept of health and wellbeing is vital in the context of health promotion.
>
> Have you thought about how health is defined and what health and wellbeing mean to you?
>
> List the various elements that you consider best describe health and wellbeing, and create a definition of health and wellbeing based on this.

The Oxford English Dictionary (2019) defines health as "the state of being free from illness or injury"; however, given the complexities surrounding health and wellbeing, this could be argued as a limited definition. In contrast, the World Health Organization (WHO) (1948) defines health as:

> …. a state of complete physical, mental and social wellbeing and not merely the absence of disease or infirmity

(Knai, 2013, p. 1)

This definition recognises that health is a holistic concept which is more in line with nursing philosophy. The approach considers the person as having many interrelating facets which include:

- biological
- sociological
- psychological
- emotional
- cultural
- spiritual.

The NMC (2018b) highlights the responsibility of nurses to consider these elements within the context of person-centred care.

The traditional medical model of health contrasts with this definition, as it is based on the principle that health is the absence of disease. The medical model measures disease and illness which has a biological origin that can be cured with a physical or chemical intervention and it positions the doctor as having more control than the patient (Scriven, 2017; Naidoo and Wills, 2009). While the origins are scientific, it could be argued that adopting a mechanical view of disease and the body is limiting and too simplistic, and risks missing out a whole-person assessment. Instead, a holistic approach to health can support the understanding of people and their behaviours. This promotes a person-centred philosophy which can enhance management and treatment of a condition.

The WHO definition of health, however, does have its critics. In 1948 it was groundbreaking, yet despite global change related to broad aspects of health in the past 60 years, this definition has not been adapted or modified. Huber *et al*. (2011) argue that the utopian principles are unachievable for most individuals and populations, and they question the feasibility of individuals to experience full and complete health and wellbeing most of the time. The WHO definition does not allow for any concept of relativity and promotes a reliance on medicalisation. This is relevant when considering chronic or terminal illness. Huber *et al.* (2011) suggest that creating a new measurement of health that is based on principles of strength, capacity to cope and psychological resilience would enhance our understanding. Focusing on the elements of quality of health, a broader and more contemporary consideration of health builds on the holistic principles of the WHO definition while moving away from the barriers associated with 'complete' health, and is in line with contemporary healthcare.

The example in *Figure 1.1* illustrates how a holistic approach to health can enhance individuals' experiences of living with a medical condition. Woolf (2018) presents a blog about promoting a holistic approach to musculoskeletal (MSK) conditions based on a new intervention arising from service user evaluation (see www.england.nhs.uk/blog/adopting-the-holistic-approach/).

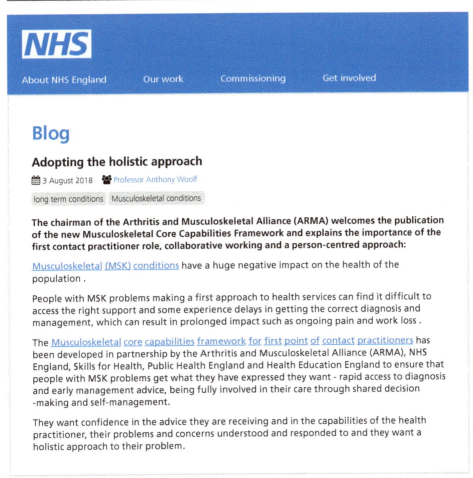

**Figure 1.1** *Excerpt from Anthony Woolf's (2018) blog on adopting a holistic approach to MSK conditions.*

Woolf highlights the value of the initial contact with a practitioner being appropriate to the individual's symptoms and level of need, rather than the traditional model of a first appointment with a general practitioner (GP). By moving away from a medical model Woolf describes how the group (ARMA) has been able to provide a collaborative, person-centred approach to avoid delay in diagnosis and management. A framework has been devised so that all practitioners working with the clients can play a meaningful role from the first point of contact, ensuring that decisions on treatment and management are shared, to promote the health and wellbeing of people with MSK conditions.

This example recognises the complexity and multifaceted nature of MSK conditions, which are typical of many long-term conditions. It illustrates that a holistic approach not only is the preferred approach of service users, but can also enhance the experience for the individual:

> They want confidence in the advice they are receiving and in the capabilities of the health practitioner, their problems and concerns understood and responded to and they want a holistic approach to their problem.
>
> (Woolf, 2018)

Interventions to promote health, such as addressing declining mobility in the ageing population, can positively impact upon individuals' level of independence as well as public funding (Bussell, 2018). This initiative therefore empowers individuals to address their health needs in relation to mobility, drawing on a range of expertise suitable to their unique circumstances. In relation to health, wellbeing and the WHO definition, this example illustrates that the traditional medical approach to treatment of a medical condition has limitations; in contrast to a more enhanced, holistic approach, which aims to achieve the best outcome. This harmonisation of skills and approaches, rather than a mechanical approach, is thought to lead to better outcomes for patients.

## 1.3 Lay concepts of health

Although the definition of health and wellbeing is complex and changeable, it is important to understand that the concept of health and wellbeing varies from person to person and that a range of factors such as an individual's previous and current experiences, profession and insights influence this. Blaxter (1995, p. 27) asserts that the crude perception of health is that medical knowledge is scientific, and that lay knowledge is "… unscientific, based on folk knowledge or individual experience".

In the UK a large-scale survey on what health meant to individuals in 1987 identified that absence of disease, physical and psychological coping and psychosocial wellbeing were key (Blaxter, cited in Thurston, 2014). Thurston (2014) explains that these findings illustrate that health from a lay perspective is multi-dimensional, adding that how health is understood varies depending on age, gender and social class of individuals. Blaxter (1995) provides the example of gender, stating that men in the survey cited health as being related to fitness and physical strength, whereas women related health to appearance and energy. While arguably stereotypical viewpoints arose from the era, the influence of many factors should be acknowledged. Nurses promote a holistic approach to enhance person-centred care and the NMC (2018a) highlights that registrants should ensure that people's physical, social and psychological needs are assessed and responded to in efforts to prevent ill health. However, Thurston (2014) warns against assuming that all healthcare professionals have the upper hand in defining health. It is therefore valuable to assess the patient's own perception on what constitutes health and wellbeing, to enhance person-centred care.

Liamputtong (2012) argues that because health and illness are socially constructed, there is an additional element of culture which influences perceptions. Taylor (2012) states that this is relevant because understanding individuals' beliefs about health arising from culture can help us to understand the associated behaviours. Consider, for example, different perceptions of tanned skin representing health and wealth in contrast to pale skin. However, it is known that prolonged sun damage or ultraviolet lights used in sunbeds can increase the risk of melanoma (Cancer Research UK, 2015). Assessing individual perceptions of health is therefore valuable to tailor the care provided in the context of health and wellbeing.

## 1.4 Defining health promotion

The term 'health promotion' was not used widely until the mid-1970s (Scriven, 2017). Until the advent of health promotion, health education was used as one strategy to improve health with a central aim to inform individuals about how to improve their health. This approach did not address wider health influences and focused on an individual's responsibility over what is within their control, rather than that of wider society and government agencies, which is outside of an individual's control (Scriven, 2017; Naidoo and Wills, 2016). The term health promotion came to global prominence through the 1986 WHO Ottawa Charter (WHO, 1986). This landmark Charter is discussed more later. The WHO defined the term health promotion as *"... the process of enabling people to increase control over, and to improve their health"* (WHO, 1986, p. 1). However, there has been, and continues to be, discussion about the concept and no single definition has been agreed upon (Whitehead, 2018).

### ACTIVITY 1.2

Consider what you have read so far in this chapter and identify ways that an individual might increase control over their health. How, as a nursing student, might you support an individual in this?

Alongside the differing opinions on how to define health promotion are the differing opinions on how health promotion can be practised and to some extent, what health promotion consists of (Scriven, 2017; Naidoo and Wills, 2016). It is important to highlight that the scope of health promotion goes beyond the role of the nurse, not only within the healthcare arena as nurses work as part of a multidisciplinary team, but also as the wider determinants of health are impacted by other groups/agencies, e.g. health and social care policy. That said, nurses are ideally placed to potentially have a significant impact on health through the principles of Making Every Contact Count (MECC) (Public Health England (PHE), 2016). The premise of MECC is using routine appointments to engage individuals in a short but effective conversation to support health and wellbeing (PHE, 2016). MECC is explored in more detail in *Chapter 6*.

Two more recent definitions of health promotion come from the National Institute for Health and Care Excellence (NICE) (2019) and Naidoo and Wills (2016), and give some direction regarding what health promotion is:

> … *giving people the information or resources they need to improve their health. As well as improving people's skills and capabilities, it can also involve changing the social and environmental conditions and systems that affect health.*
>
> (NICE, 2019)

> *Health promotion is a range of activities and interventions to enable people to take greater control over their health. Activities may be directed at individuals, families, communities or whole populations.*
>
> (Naidoo and Wills, 2016, p. 125)

These two definitions identify that actions taken for health promotion focus on informing, empowering and enabling. This resonates with the three strategies outlined by the WHO Ottawa Charter (WHO, 1986) of advocate, enable and mediate. This highlights that although the definitions here are different, the golden thread of improving health and supporting individuals to have control of their health connects them.

> **ACTIVITY 1.3**
>
> Consider the role of a specialist nurse who works in coronary care. What health promotion activities or interventions could they use in daily practice?

Significant events such as recovery from an acute medical emergency, or experiencing a life event such as pregnancy and birth offer nurses opportunities for health promotion. Naidoo and Wills (2009) state that health promotion seeks to evoke behaviour change and health education can support this. Health education is structured and takes a planned approach to providing information about health, aiming to change an individual's behaviour (Naidoo and Wills, 2009) and is closely linked to the concept of health literacy. In broad terms, health literacy refers to improving access to and understanding of health-related information, achieved through a variety of means including, for example, supporting an individual to have the confidence to take action to improve their health (WHO, 1998). This concept is explored more fully in *Chapter 6*.

Health education is, of course, not as simple as providing information (Whitehead, 2018). There is the potential for health education to be viewed as one-sided, because it is delivered by the nurse and received by the client. This is not the aim of health education; rather it is to be a conversation that leaves the decision to act, or not; to change behaviour, or not, to the individual (Naidoo and Wills, 2009). As a nurse, you need to consider what your client already understands about their health, how best to promote an evidence-based discussion and how to engage and empower the client to make an informed choice for themselves. Exploration and recognition of an individual's attitudes, values and beliefs support a person-centred conversation (Marshall, Baston and Hall, 2019). To be effective, health promotion should empower individuals, groups or communities (Whitehead, 2018) and this can be evident in a variety of scenarios.

> **ACTIVITY 1.4**
>
> What actions could you take to ensure you provide personalised health education to a client in your care?
>
> Consider: the environment, the person, active listening skills and how you might supportively signpost the client at the end of your discussion.

Different approaches to health promotion are likely to continue to emerge due to the shifting nature of health and the environment. The seriousness of the climate crisis is being realised, new illnesses continue to emerge and political policies change as new governments gain power. Health promotion is responsive, reflecting advances, discoveries and challenges in the field. For example, health promotion activities may include emergency response planning for disasters linked to extreme weather, the prevention of communicable diseases – which has become increasingly challenging with the accessibility of international travel – or strategies that tackle loneliness, which is an increasing social problem. Similarly, modern health promotion strategies may make use of social media as a tool to disseminate health information, which was not feasible just a decade ago.

Future nurses will be expected to have a clear role in health promotion. PHE (2013) called for each individual nurse to be a "health promoting practitioner". While there are specialist health promotion practitioners, it is each nurse's responsibility to promote health. This is clear in the NMC's *Future Nurse* (NMC, 2018a) *Standards of Proficiency* document, which defines the necessary skills and attributes required of nurses upon registration.

There is considerable scope for nurses to positively impact health and wellbeing, because they provide care across the lifespan. While there are numerous opportunities to promote health with each client/nurse interaction, it is essential that this is done in inclusive and accessible ways. In 2016 the Royal College of Nursing (RCN) carried out a project to identify how commissioners and public health service planners and designers viewed and valued the role of nurses in improving public health (RCN, 2016). One of the key findings highlighted by the RCN was that nurses were considered more approachable than some other healthcare practitioners (HCPs) (RCN, 2016). This demonstrates the pivotal role nurses have within the diverse group of practitioners that support health promotion.

> **ACTIVITY 1.5**
>
> What does health promotion mean to you?
>
> Consider what you have read so far and any clinical practice experience you may have had in health promotion and write down what this means to you. You may want to discuss this with a fellow nursing student and compare your thoughts.

## 1.5 Public health

The NMC (2018a) highlights that the role of the registered nurse in promoting health and preventing ill health is supported by active engagement with public health. Within a nursing context public health is associated with principles of health promotion, health education and public health and the prevention of ill health (NMC, 2018a; RCN, 2019). To enhance and protect health and wellbeing are common aims within nursing practice. This section will explore some of the principles of public health and its application to contemporary practice.

The Faculty of Public Health (2016, p. 2) defines public health as:

> …the science and art of promoting and protecting health and wellbeing, preventing ill-health and prolonging life through the organised efforts of society.

The definition illustrates that the practice of public health is broad, holistic and that many factors contribute in the understanding of problems to find solutions. The practice of public health therefore embraces numerous means, working with a range of professional bodies, services and infrastructures to empower a healthy community. Public health is a positive global step working towards equilibrium to enhance individual, community and population wellbeing. The WHO (2019a) identifies that attention to all aspects of health and wellbeing, rather than the eradication of certain conditions, promotes the elements of public health.

The origins of public health within the UK were first recognised with the desire to improve environmental conditions to improve health outcomes. In the nineteenth century the sanitation of drinking water and safe disposal of sewage impacted positively on the health of the nation. McKeown's studies (1976, cited in Lee and Collin, 2005) illustrated that in contrast to previous beliefs about health, mortality rates did not reduce due to antibiotic therapy or vaccination programmes; instead it was improved living conditions, including sanitation and nutrition, that impacted most upon mortality rates. While this argument has since been contested, the fundamental principle is that medical advances have less impact than social improvement within public health.

Health expectancy in the past century has increased significantly, with modern-day mortality and morbidity associated increasingly with non-communicable diseases rather than the previous primary cause of infectious diseases (McMichael and Beaglehole, 2009; Thurston, 2014; RCN, 2019). Knowledge and evidence related to public health has identified that social inequalities found within modern society have created health inequalities among poorer groups. Added to this is the acknowledgement that complex influences on health and wellbeing can determine the health of individuals and populations more than the actual state of physical health (Liamputtong, 2012). These determinants of health include a range of personal, environmental, social, economic and cultural factors. Wilkinson and Marmot's (2003) report and, more recently, *Health Equity in England: the Marmot Review 10 years on* (Marmot, 2020) illustrate that people's health is strongly influenced by lifestyle and living and working conditions, advocating for health policy to address this. McMichael and Beaglehole (2009) highlight that these health inequalities are supported by political, social and behavioural determinants and it is vital that these are understood and acted upon to effectively influence the change required. Environmental factors can also influence population health, illustrating the complexity surrounding current public health issues.

### ACTIVITY 1.6

Read more about inequalities of health by accessing one of the following key reports:
- *Independent Inquiry into Inequalities in Health*, also known as the Acheson Report (Acheson, 1988; available at bit.ly/1-6IH)
- *Fair Society, Healthy Lives*, also known as the Marmot Review (Marmot, 2010; available at bit.ly/1-6FS)
- *Health Equity in England: the Marmot Review 10 years on* (Marmot, 2020; available at bit.ly/1-6HE).

These reports highlight a range of recommendations related to social inequalities and health.

The science related to public health is measured through epidemiological studies. These are in-depth analyses of the distribution and determinants of diseases and injuries in human populations, and form the basis of all decision-making on public health issues (Hubley and Copeman, 2013; Gillam, Yates and Padmanabhan, 2012). A common measurement used is prevalence. The prevalence rate enables understanding of attributes during a specific time interval. This can include disease, infections and long-term conditions. Changing health patterns may be attributed to a number of factors including health screening, medical interventions and lifestyle factors such as alcohol and tobacco consumption, obesity and a reduction in physical activity. The Global Burden of Disease study illustrated that poor diet and smoking were two behaviours that contributed most to the number of deaths in the UK (Newton, 2015). In developed countries today the most significant threat to people's health is associated with lifestyle behaviours, requiring responsive public health prioritisation to promote and improve the health of the nation (Lock and Sim, 2009).

> ### ACTIVITY 1.7
>
> Consider the example of sedentary behaviour and reduced physical activity to demonstrate the points raised here. Think about political, social, behavioural and environmental influences that may lead to a reduction in physical activity within population groups.
>
> Create lists using political, social, behavioural and environmental elements as headings to guide you.

Public health makes efforts to not only understand the problem but also combat it through prevention or reduction of harm through interagency working (Carr, Unwin and Pless-Mulloli, 2007). These include government agencies, local authorities, executive agencies, service leadership and charitable organisations; see *Table 1.1* for examples.

**Table 1.1** *Agencies in public health and examples*

| Agency | Example |
| --- | --- |
| Government agencies | Food Standards Agency |
| Local authorities | Sexual health clinics for the local population |
| Executive agencies | Public Health Wales |
| Service leadership | NHS England |
| Charitable organisations | Action on Smoking and Health (ASH) Wales |

Utilising the example of childhood obesity, solutions are widely postulated. Despite the complexities surrounding childhood obesity, Ebbeling, Pawlak and Ludwig (2002) call for a commonsense approach. They discuss the virtues of family-based and school-based interventions in contrast to pharmacological or surgical approaches. In exploring this modern public health phenomenon, they highlight that sedentary lifestyle, reckless food advertising and environmental restrictions on play impact upon the issue. A review by Karnik and Kanekar (2012) illustrated that population-based approaches to increase physical activity and healthy diet were successful, enhancing sustainability and longevity in solutions.

Sustainable approaches to public health are currently key, both globally and in the UK and *The NHS Long Term Plan* (NHS, 2019) has identified ten key priorities for public health which reflect this:
1. Prevention
2. Smoking
3. Obesity and type 2 diabetes
4. Diet and alcohol

5. Antimicrobial resistance and vaccines
6. Cancer
7. Mental health
8. Air pollution
9. Children and maternity care
10. Gambling.

Given the broad spectrum of population-based issues, the solution is often unlikely to lie with one 'treatment' or medicalised approach. Public health draws on knowledge underpinned by sociology, psychology, health economics, epidemiology, management and leadership. This 'whole systems' approach accepts that health issues are complex and that the solutions are, therefore, multifaceted and often include fiscal policy and legislative and social initiatives, in addition to specific condition prevention measures (Carr, Unwin and Pless-Mulloli, 2007). It is important to recognise that not only individuals, but each population is unique in its needs and the subsequent approaches required. In designing interventions for community or population groups it is important to understand that a public health approach is concerned with the 'greater good' for society or populations rather than the individual. The individual often benefits from public health programmes; however, at times when faced with large numbers the majority benefit, but not necessarily every individual (Somerville, Kumaran and Anderson, 2012). Many public health activities are therefore targeted at specific groups or populations, but some public health services also include the provision of services to prevent disease within the entire population, for example through vaccination programmes (RCN, 2019).

Nurses often provide this type of intervention; it is, therefore, important that we recognise the considerable impact of public health practice (Coles and Porter, 2008). Public Health England (2019) developed the "All our Health" framework to support all nurses and healthcare professionals in the use of their knowledge, skills and relationships to prevent illness, protect health and promote wellbeing. The framework advocates that frontline staff can approach this in three ways: being proactive to prevent illness and promote health, working alongside individuals and communities to inform choices, and utilisation of MECC (PHE, 2016).

While public health is often associated with the eradication of disease, as seen in vaccination programmes both globally and nationally, knowledge and understanding of the full spectrum of health and wellbeing are fundamental principles of public health action. Sustained activities to enhance and strengthen public health capacity, as well as the provision of conditions where populations can live in a healthy way, are demonstrable in various public health initiatives. These aim to maintain health, improve health and wellbeing or prevent health deterioration. Often these organised efforts are associated with improving health outcomes for targeted groups. In the media, this is often demonstrated with pandemic disease eradication by a range of groups in poorer nations. A public health approach can involve addressing societal health inequalities by tackling wider determinants of health and wellbeing, as well as protecting the population from hazards to health. In addition, fiscal and legislative changes can have positive impacts. For examples of these see *Table 1.2*. Underlying the theories and methods of these three paradigms is their contribution to health protection.

> **ACTIVITY 1.8**
>
> Access information about the key areas for public health identified in *The NHS Long Term Plan*. Select two areas and make bullet points on the rationale and purpose of the targeted approach, with a specific practice area in mind.

## 1.6 The World Health Organization and health promotion

The World Health Organization (WHO) is the directing and coordinating authority on international health for the United Nations (UN) (WHO, 2019b). The WHO works in numerous ways to reduce health inequalities, build healthier futures for everyone across the globe and combat disease (WHO, 2019c). The diverse work the WHO engages in can be read about in more detail at www.who.int/about.

Global health promotion is a fundamental component of the work the WHO undertakes. This was initiated in the landmark Ottawa Charter (WHO, 1986), launched at the first WHO international conference on health promotion. It was at the inaugural conference in 1986 where the mandate for advocating the promotion of health and supporting nations to initiate health promotion strategies was placed upon the WHO and other international organisations (WHO, 1986). While the Ottawa Charter is viewed as the key strategic document that elevated health promotion as a concept, preceding publications provided the necessary foundations for the Charter to take centre stage, including: the WHO constitution (WHO, 1948), specifically the way it defined health in positive terms; the Lalonde Report (Lalonde, 1974); and the Declaration of Alma-Ata (WHO, 1978; Potvin and Jones, 2011).

The Charter identifies that optimising health is not just an individual's responsibility; it is that of wider society too. Moreover, it also identifies that the responsibility of health promotion is not limited to the healthcare sector. In order to generate the most conducive environment for health promotion, the Charter recommends three strategies for health promoters to adopt:

- **Advocate** – this relates to taking a holistic view when advocating for health, encouraging factors at both an individual (e.g. cultural, behavioural) and societal (e.g. political, environmental) level to be optimised
- **Enable** – this emphasises the need to minimise inequalities in health and optimise good health for all
- **Mediate** – this outlines the importance of health promotion action to take a multilevel and strategic approach.

The Charter states that for health promotion action to be effective, it must be meaningful to the individuals, societal groups and cultures that it seeks to help. Therefore, five action areas were identified as ways to support health:
1. Building healthy public policy, at all sectors and levels of government
2. Creating supportive environments, to improve living and working conditions

3. Strengthening community action in priority setting and in strategies
4. Developing personal skills, through education for health and life skills
5. Reorienting health services towards health promotion.

The action areas emphasise the WHO message that the responsibility to maintain good health is not simply for each individual to bear; rather it is essential that wider society and societal systems at a macro level support health and offer a conducive environment to promote health. We will return to these themes throughout the book.

### ACTIVITY 1.9

Access the Ottawa Charter at bit.ly/1-9OC and read more about the five Action Areas. Focus on 'Create Supportive Environments' and consider ways in which hospitals have become health-promoting for both those who work in them and members of the public accessing services.

The Charter is regarded as the most influential global health promotion movement (Whitehead, 2018) and cited as the "foundational document" of health promotion by Potvin and Jones (2011, p. 244). Thompson, Watson and Tilford (2018) cite the Charter as pivotal in changing the conversation around health promotion from an individual's responsibility and how individuals are affected, to identifying how societal systems such as government, schools and environments can promote health. This is in part attributed to the Charter presenting a positive definition of health (Potvin and Jones, 2011) and the importance of preserving and creating health, moving the focus away from disease. While the Ottawa Charter is three decades old, it is still highly influential in health promotion practices today (Naidoo and Wills, 2016; Thompson, Watson and Tilford, 2018). The five action areas were reconfirmed in the Jakarta Declaration on leading health promotion into the 21st century in 1997 (WHO, 2009) and Naidoo and Wills (2016) contend that the action areas provide a framework for contemporary health promotion practice.

### ACTIVITY 1.10

Explore the WHO's work through their website (www.who.int). Consider choosing a health topic by country to focus on an area that interests you.

Since 1986 there have been eight further international conferences on health promotion setting out strategic pathways to achieve global health goals. More recent programmes of work to support health globally include the UN's Millennium Development Goals (MDGs), eight goals with defined targets set in 2000 which were to be achieved by 2015 (UN, 2015). The unified work of nations resulted in some of the MDGs being fully or partially realised and these results are described as remarkable; however, the most vulnerable remain at risk of poverty, ill health and social exclusion (UN, 2015). The MDGs address some wider determinants of health but also contemporary health challenges, for example promoting gender equality (UN, 2015).

Building on the MDGs the UN set out the Sustainable Development Goals (SDGs) in 2015; seventeen goals reflecting substantial contemporary global challenges to be achieved by 2030 with the aim to "leave no one behind" (UN, 2019a). The SDGs are a call to action for all countries, not just developed countries as with the MDGs. The SDGs require action at all levels, described as global, local and people action (UN, 2019b). While the SDGs require simultaneous multilevel action in order to meet the considerable number of targets, the role of the individual is clear, whether they are a nurse or not. The SDGs reflect the intersectional approach to support and promote health set out in the five action areas of the Ottawa Charter (WHO, 1986).

### ACTIVITY 1.11

Read Sustainable Development Goal 3: Ensure healthy lives and promote wellbeing for all at all ages, available at bit.ly/1-11SDG. Looking at the information relating to maternal health, investigate some health promotion activities that could support the areas requiring development.

The information presented in this chapter has highlighted the broad remit of health promotion, health education and public health. They are multifaceted and often interlink and overlap within various activities in tackling one broad issue. Use *Activity 1.12* to confirm your understanding of the various elements.

### ACTIVITY 1.12

Obesity is a growing epidemic within the UK. Consider which paradigm (health promotion/health education/public health) each activity is most suited to in the context of tackling obesity across the life course. Further reading to support you in this exercise is:
A. *Sugar tax revenue helps tackle childhood obesity* (at bit.ly/1-12A)
B. *Final design of consistent nutritional labelling system given green light* (at bit.ly/1-12B)
C. *The Education (Nutritional Standards for School Lunches) (England) Regulations 2006* (at bit.ly/1-12C)
D. *Health matters: getting every adult active every day* (at bit.ly/1-12D)
E. *Easy ways to make lunchboxes healthier* (at bit.ly/1-12E)
F. *Obesity UK website* (at bit.ly/1-12F)
G. NICE CG43: *Obesity prevention* (at bit.ly/1-12G)
H. WHO: *Exclusive breastfeeding to reduce the risk of childhood overweight and obesity* (at bit.ly/1-12H)
I. WHO: *Fiscal policies for diet and the prevention of noncommunicable diseases* (at bit.ly/1-12I)

*Table 1.2* gives the answers to *Activity 1.12* and demonstrates that several of the areas draw on public health, health promotion and health education, whereas others have a specific focus: public health underpins items A–C and E; D, F and G are examples of Health Education; and areas C, F and H are examples of health promotion. As you will see, C and F are underpinned by two paradigms.

**Table 1.2** Health promotion, health education and public health integration that support health protection

| Area | Activity | Public health | Health promotion | Health education |
|---|---|:---:|:---:|:---:|
| A. Fiscal | Part of the WHO global action plan for the prevention and control of non-communicable diseases 2013–20: Introduction of Soft Drinks Industry Levy (SDIL) to encourage soft drink manufacturers to reduce sugar content through a government initiative to tackle childhood obesity | ✔ | | |
| B. Non-mandatory ministerial policy | Voluntary front of pack nutrition labelling in an easily recognisable form to help purchasers determine which products are healthier and which are not | ✔ | | |
| C. Legislative | UK government has introduced nutritional standards for school lunches, including regulations that fruit and vegetables are offered as part of every school meal | ✔ | ✔ | |
| D. Environment | PHE supports the prioritisation of developing roads, including re-allocation of road spaces to support individuals to walk and cycle, increasing their daily physical activity | ✔ | | |
| E. Education sector | Local school education to children and parents on healthy lunchboxes using Change4life | | | ✔ |

| | | | | |
|---|---|---|---|---|
| F. Charity | Obesity UK provides a mutual support group and link for individuals with a raised BMI and healthcare organisations that provide evidence-based weight management services | | ✓ | ✓ |
| G. Healthcare evidence | Resources outline how a range of stakeholders support clients to increase physical activity levels and improve dietary intakes amongst targeted populations, e.g. NICE CG43. *Obesity prevention* | | | ✓  |
| H. HCPs | Midwives provide support on exclusive breastfeeding to avoid inappropriate complementary feeding practices, such as early introduction of complementary foods, that could result in unhealthy weight gain | | ✓ | |

### KEY LEARNING POINTS

Three key points to take away from *Chapter 1*:
- ☑ Health promotion, health education and public health are expansive, multifaceted and responsive to contemporary healthcare.
- ☑ Health promotion, health education and public health often interlink and overlap to tackle one broad issue.
- ☑ Nurses have an essential role in supporting the advancement of the health of individuals through the areas of health promotion, health education and public health.

# REFERENCES

Acheson, D. (1988) *Independent Inquiry into Inequalities in Health Report*. Available at: https://assets.publishing.service.gov.uk/government/uploads/system/uploads/attachment_data/file/265503/ih.pdf (accessed 6 May 2020)

Blaxter, M. (1995) 'What is health?' In Davey, B., Gray, A. and Seale, C. (eds) *Health and Disease: a reader*, 2nd edition. Open University Press.

Bussell, G. (2018) Considerations for weight loss and activity in the over 60s. *Journal of Community Nursing,* **32(4):** 57–61.

Cancer Research UK (2015) *Risks and causes of melanoma*. Available at: www.cancerresearchuk.org/about-cancer/melanoma/risks-causes (accessed 6 May 2020)

Carr, S., Unwin, N. and Pless-Mulloli, T. (2007) *An Introduction to Public Health and Epidemiology*, 2nd edition. McGraw-Hill Education.

Coles, L. and Porter, E. (eds) (2008) *Public Health Skills: a practical guide for nurses and public health practitioners*. Blackwell Publishing.

Ebbeling, C., Pawlak, D. and Ludwig, D. (2002) Childhood obesity: public-health crisis, common sense cure. *The Lancet,* **360(9331):** 473–82.

Faculty of Public Health (2016) *Good Public Health Practice Framework Short Guide*. Available at: www.fph.org.uk/media/1305/short-guide_good-public-health-practice_april-2016.pdf (accessed 6 May 2020)

Gillam, S., Yates, J. and Padmanabhan, B. (eds) (2012) *Essential Public Health: theory and practice*, 2nd edition. Cambridge University Press.

Huber, M., Knottnerus, A., Green, L., *et al*. (2011) How should we define health? *BMJ,* **343:** d4163.

Hubley, J. and Copeman, J. (2013) *Practical Health Promotion,* 2nd edition. Polity Press.

Karnik, S. and Kanekar, A. (2012) Childhood obesity: a global public health crisis. *International Journal of Preventative Medicine*, **3(1):** 1–7.

Knai, C. (2013) 'What is Public Health?' In Thornbory, G. (ed.) *Public Health Nursing: a textbook for health visitors, school nurses and occupational health nurses*. Wiley-Blackwell.

Lalonde, M. (1974) *A New Perspective on the Health of Canadians: a working document*. Available at: www.phac-aspc.gc.ca/ph-sp/pdf/perspect-eng.pdf (accessed 6 May 2020)

Lee, K. and Collin, J. (eds) (2005) *Global Change and Health*. Open University Press.

Liamputtong, P. (2012) 'Health, illness and well-being: an introduction.' In Liamputtong, P., Fanany, R. and Verrinder, G. (eds) *Health, Illness and Well-being: perspectives and social determinants*. Oxford University Press.

Lock, K. and Sim, F. (2009) 'Public health in the United Kingdom.' In Beaglehole, R. and Bonita, R. (eds) *Global Public Health: a new era,* 2nd edition. Oxford University Press.

Marmot, M. (2010) *Fair Society, Healthy Lives*. Available at: www.parliament.uk/documents/fair-society-healthy-lives-full-report.pdf (accessed 6 May 2020)

Marmot, M. (2020) *Health Equity in England: the Marmot review 10 years on*. Institute of Health Equity. Available at: www.health.org.uk/sites/default/files/upload/publications/2020/Health%20Equity%20in%20England_The%20Marmot%20Review%2010%20Years%20On_full%20report.pdf (accessed 6 May 2020)

Marshall, J., Baston, H. and Hall, J. (2019) *Midwifery Essentials: public health*. Elsevier.

McMichael, A. and Beaglehole, R. (2009) 'The global context for public health.' In Beaglehole, R. and Bonita, R. (eds) *Global Public Health: a new era,* 2nd edition. Oxford University Press.

Naidoo, J. and Wills, J. (2009) *Foundations for Health Promotion*, 3rd edition. Elsevier.

Naidoo, J. and Wills, J. (2016) *Foundations for Health Promotion*, 4th edition. Elsevier.

National Institute for Health and Care Excellence (2019) *Glossary*. Available at: www.nice.org.uk/Glossary?letter=H (accessed 20 May 2020)

Newton, J. (2015) *The Burden of Disease and What it Means in England*. Available at: https://publichealthmatters.blog.gov.uk/2015/09/15/the-burden-of-disease-and-what-it-means-in-england/ (accessed 6 May 2020)

NHS (2019) *The NHS Long Term Plan*. Available at: www.longtermplan.nhs.uk/wp-content/uploads/2019/08/nhs-long-term-plan-version-1.2.pdf (accessed 6 May 2020)

Nursing and Midwifery Council (2018a) *Future Nurse: standards of proficiency for registered nurses*. Available at: www.nmc.org.uk/standards/standards-for-nurses/standards-of-proficiency-for-registered-nurses (accessed 6 May 2020)

Nursing and Midwifery Council (2018b) *The Code: professional standards of practice and behaviour for nurses, midwives and nursing associates*. Available at: www.nmc.org.uk/standards/code (accessed 6 May 2020)

Oxford English Dictionary (2019) *Health*. Available at: www.lexico.com/definition/health (accessed 6 May 2020)

Potvin, L. and Jones, C. (2011) Twenty-five years after the Ottawa Charter: the critical role of health promotion for public health. *Canadian Journal of Public Health*, **102(4)**: 244–8. Available at: https://link.springer.com/article/10.1007/BF03404041 (accessed 6 May 2020)

Public Health England (2013) *Nursing and Midwifery Contribution to Public Health*. Available at: www.gov.uk/government/publications/nursing-and-midwifery-contribution-to-public-health (accessed 6 May 2020)

Public Health England (2016) *Making Every Contact Count (MECC): consensus statement*. Available at: www.gov.uk/government/publications/making-every-contact-count-mecc-practical-resources (accessed 6 May 2020)

Public Health England (2019) *All Our Health: about the framework*. Available at: www.gov.uk/government/publications/all-our-health-about-the-framework (accessed 6 May 2020)

Royal College of Nursing (2016) *Nurses 4 Public Health: promote, prevent and protect. The value and contribution of nursing to public health in the UK: final report*. Available at: www.rcn.org.uk/-/media/royal-college-of-nursing/documents/clinical-topics/public-health/nurses-4-public-health.pdf?la=en&hash=BC9137D960B0808551FE6E16986A7B71 (accessed 6 May 2020)

Royal College of Nursing (2019) *Public Health*. Available at: www.rcn.org.uk/clinical-topics/public-health (accessed 6 May 2020)

Scriven, A. (2017) *Ewles & Simnett's Promoting Health: a practical guide*, 7th edition. Elsevier.

Somerville, M., Kumaran, K. and Anderson, R. (2012) *Public Health and Epidemiology at a Glance*. Wiley-Blackwell.

Taylor, S. (2012) 'Human genetics and inheritance: biological, social, cultural and environmental perspectives.' In Liamputtong, P., Fanany, R. and Verrinder, G. (eds) *Health, Illness and Well-being: perspectives and social determinants*. Oxford University Press.

Thompson, S., Watson, M. and Tilford, S. (2018) The Ottawa Charter 30 years on: still an important standard for health promotion. *International Journal of Health Promotion and Education*, **56(2)**: 73–84. Available at: www.tandfonline.com/doi/abs/10.1080/14635240.2017.1415765 (accessed 6 May 2020)

Thurston, M. (2014) *Key Themes in Public Health*. Routledge.

United Nations (2015) *The Millennium Development Goals Report 2015*. Available at: www.un.org/millenniumgoals/2015_MDG_Report/pdf/MDG%202015%20rev%20(July%201).pdf (accessed 6 May 2020)

United Nations (2019a) *Sustainable Development Goals*. Available at: www.un.org/sustainabledevelopment (accessed 6 May 2020)

United Nations (2019b) *The Sustainable Development Agenda: a decade of action*. Available at: www.un.org/sustainabledevelopment/development-agenda (accessed 6 May 2020)

Whitehead, D. (2018) Exploring health promotion and health education in nursing. *Nursing Standard*, **33(8)**: 38–44.

Wilkinson, R. and Marmot, M. (eds) (2003) *Social Determinants of Health: the solid facts*, 2nd edition. WHO. Available at: www.euro.who.int/__data/assets/pdf_file/0005/98438/e81384.pdf (accessed 6 May 2020)

World Health Organization (1948) *WHO Definition of Health*. Preamble to the Constitution of WHO as adopted by the International Health Conference, New York, 19 June – 22 July 1946; signed on 22 July 1946 by the representatives of 61 States (Official Records of WHO, no. 2, p. 100) and entered into force on 7 April 1948. Available at: http://apps.who.int/gb/bd/PDF/bd47/EN/constitution-en.pdf?ua=1 (accessed 6 May 2020)

World Health Organization (1978) *Declaration of Alma-Ata*. Available at: www.who.int/publications/almaata_declaration_en.pdf (accessed 6 May 2020)

World Health Organization (1986) *Ottawa Charter for Health Promotion*. Available at: www.euro.who.int/__data/assets/pdf_file/0004/129532/Ottawa_Charter.pdf?ua=1 (accessed 6 May 2020)

World Health Organization (1998) *Health Literacy*. Available at: www.who.int/healthpromotion/health-literacy/en (accessed 6 May 2020)

World Health Organization (2009) *Milestones in Health Promotion: statements from global conferences*. Available at: www.who.int/healthpromotion/Milestones_Health_Promotion_05022010.pdf (accessed 6 May 2020)

World Health Organization (2019a) *Public Health Services*. Available at: www.euro.who.int/en/health-topics/Health-systems/public-health-services (accessed 6 May 2020)

World Health Organization (2019b) *Our Values*. Available at: www.who.int/about/who-we-are/our-values (accessed 6 May 2020)

World Health Organization (2019c) *About WHO*. Available at: www.who.int/about (accessed 6 May 2020)

Woolf, A. (2018) *Adopting the Holistic Approach* blog. Available at: www.england.nhs.uk/blog/adopting-the-holistic-approach (accessed 6 May 2020)

# Chapter 2
# Behaviour change: theories, models and approaches

Stephen Scott

> **LEARNING OUTCOMES**
>
> When you have finished this chapter, you should be able to:
>
> **2.1** Discuss the nature of behavioural change and health promotion
>
> **2.2** Identify the health behaviours that need to change to promote health
>
> **2.3** Outline the mechanisms that support behavioural change
>
> **2.4** Identify and address barriers to change
>
> **2.5** Describe what change process is suitable at which point in the patient's journey.

## 2.1 Introduction

Behavioural change theory and practice is influenced by a range of academic disciplines including sociology, health education, management and health psychology (Michie, Atkins and West, 2014). It is focused on identifying targets for change, developing skills and mechanisms that support people through change and identifying stages people go through as they change. Behaviour change theory provides a scientific underpinning to nurses' health promotion practice, while placing the patient at the heart of all interventions (Murdaugh, Parsons and Pender, 2019).

This chapter will systematically take you through the most prominent theories and models of behavioural change that support nursing practice. The approaches discussed focus on creating changes in behaviour to enhance the health and wellbeing of our patients.

> ### ACTIVITY 2.1
>
> Consider the focus of behavioural change in the following range of professions. What outcomes are the professionals targeting?
> - Probation worker
> - Teacher
> - Team GB hockey coach

You may have identified that probation workers focus on reducing reoffending rates or increasing social inclusion, teachers focus on promoting authentic learning or maximising pupil achievement and in sport, a coach is likely to wish to optimise the team's competitive advantage.

> ### ACTIVITY 2.2
>
> Now consider the focus of behavioural change in nursing.

Behavioural change in nursing practice is primarily focused on modifying behaviour to improve the health, wellbeing and functioning of the target population. Behavioural change is central to health promotion. It focuses on moving patients away from health-defeating behaviours and towards health-enhancing behaviours (Cragg, Davies and MacDowall, 2013). In contrast to the medical model that was introduced in *Chapter 1*, Murdaugh, Parsons and Pender (2019) assert that nursing is a process focused on building health in our patients and wider society. Health promotion is, therefore, at the heart of nursing practice.

> ### ACTIVITY 2.3
>
> Spend a few moments considering how a focus on health promotion fits with your perceptions of nursing practice, before you move on.

## 2.2 Determinants of health

Identifying factors that determine a greater likelihood of poor health gives us an indication of the influence we may need to apply to promote health and wellbeing and reduce the burden that ill health creates in society. Dahlgren and Whitehead (1991) focus our attention towards the "determinants of health". Their model supports the development of health promotion initiatives in relation to broad population need, helping us recognise both at-risk groups and factors correlated with poor health that are amenable to change. These factors include:

- fixed personal predisposing factors, such as sex, age, ethnic group and hereditary factors
- individual 'lifestyle' factors, including behaviours such as smoking, alcohol use and physical activity
- social and community networks, including family and wider social circles

- living and working conditions, such as access and opportunities regarding access to jobs, housing, education and welfare services
- general socioeconomic, cultural and environmental conditions, including factors such as disposable income, taxation and availability of work.

These factors combine to create what the authors call the core "determinants of health". Dahlgren and Whitehead (1991) give a visual map of these determinants of health to help clinicians identify the key determinants associated with health burdens (see *Figure 2.1*).

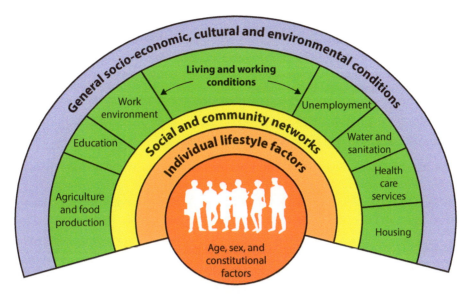

**Figure 2.1** *The Dahlgren–Whitehead rainbow. Reproduced by kind permission from: Dahlgren, G. and Whitehead, M. (1991) Policies and Strategies to Promote Social Equity in Health. Stockholm, Sweden: Institute for Futures Studies.*

*Case study 2.1* introduces the Bevan family. The Bevan family help us understand the main determinants of health. They also highlight three different focuses for health promotion, recognising the distinction between primary, secondary and tertiary health promotion needs and processes.

- At a primary level the nurse may focus on promoting health in the whole population, including those who presently have no signs of illness (Rhys)
- At a secondary level the focus is on preventing deterioration in those with signs of illness who would benefit from intervention (David).
- At a tertiary level the focus shifts to preserving functioning in people with long-term or enduring conditions (Lewis) (Naidoo and Wills, 2016).

> **CASE STUDY 2.1  THE BEVAN FAMILY**
>
> Rhys Bevan is 27 and lives in a city; he works in the finance industry, he is well and enjoying his time in the city but eats mainly fast food and drinks alcohol most evenings. He weighs 16st 2lb (102kg) and is 5ft 10in (178cm) tall. David, Rhys's uncle, has undertaken genetic testing which identified a marker for Alzheimer's dementia. David lives alone; he has begun to slow down and occasionally forgets important dates and faces. He retired 6 months ago at the age of 60 after a career in the mining industry followed by labouring roles. He has few friends but continues to socialise in the local community social club. Lewis is 65; he is Rhys's father. He took over a tenant hill farm from his father at 13 years of age and lives in the same farmhouse in a very rural setting with his wife Margaret, who now largely manages their farm. Lewis has been supported by the local memory day clinic for the past 3 years following deterioration in his memory and functioning, which led to a provisional diagnosis of Alzheimer's disease. Lewis still enjoys feeding the cows and identifying stock for future breeding.

To understand the determinants of health in *Case study 2.1* we need to understand the factors that are important to the health of this family.

Dementia can have a major impact on a person's care needs and their functional capacity (Prince *et al.*, 2015). It has been identified as a major health burden to our society in the Prime Minister's 2020 Challenge on Dementia: Implementation Plan (DHSC, 2016) and the Dementia 2020 Challenge Progress Review Part 1 (DHSC, 2019). Both reports highlight the significant cost of dementia onset in terms of quality of life (QOL), state financial burden and health resource usage. This burden has been reviewed in detail and Heginbotham and Newbigging (2013) identify it as a central concern for health promotion services. In 2018 the Alzheimer's Association evaluated the national statistics identifying a UK population of 537 097 diagnosed cases of dementia and estimating this will rise to well over one million by 2025 (Alzheimer's Research UK, 2018).

However, knowing these facts relating to the burden of dementia offers little guidance in relation to reducing health, wellbeing and cost-based burdens. To reduce the health burden here, we need to identify the factors that might influence the health outcomes for members of our society and develop strategies to address these. Sociologists have focused on mining sociodemographic data to identify and understand differences in health outcomes between populations so we can uncover the main factors that determine good health outcomes. The Marmot Report (Marmot, 2010) and the subsequent review (Marmot, 2020), which is addressed in detail in *Chapter 3*, was instrumental in refocusing health promotion towards inequalities in health as a mechanism to identify protective factors as well as behaviours that may damage health. Public Health England, the Public Health Observatory for Wales, the Public Health Agency in Northern Ireland and the Scottish Public Health Observatory all gather statistical data to help identify health discrepancies and to understand differences in health between populations. This data informs our understanding of health-enhancing processes and identifies targets for action.

A major study evaluating factors associated with the onset of dementia estimated that up to a third of cases of dementia could be attributable to determinants of health that would be amenable to midlife interventions (Norton *et al.*, 2014). These factors are explored in detail below. Being able to identify factors that are associated with health outcomes, otherwise known as "determinants of health", allows us to target our attempts to reduce the health burden on our society as a whole by preserving functioning at a primary, secondary and tertiary level (Cragg, Davies and MacDowall, 2013).

> **ACTIVITY 2.4**
>
> Based on your reading so far, review the Bevan family (*Case study 2.1*) to identify determinants of health that may be targeted to promote better outcomes for all. Next, consider each member of the family to identify the need for any primary, secondary or tertiary interventions.

There is no evidence that Rhys has 'personal predisposing factors' in the form of genetic links for cardiovascular disease, but in relation to Alzheimer's he may have a genetic predisposition which represents a fixed determinant of health. In addition, gender appears to have an influence on dementia prevalence, with men having a lesser incidence of dementia overall. There is a higher overall prevalence of dementia in women but a higher risk of vascular dementia in men who experience cardiovascular disease profiles (Prince *et al.*, 2014). As a male, Rhys therefore has a reduced risk of dementia overall but he has a higher risk of vascular dementia. Rhys's 'lifestyle factors', however, also place him at greater risk of vascular dementia, cardiovascular disease and dementia overall (NICE, 2014; NICE, 2015). The lifestyle determinants underpinning all three conditions are alcohol intake, diet and exercise levels (NICE, 2015). National health promotion guidance for dementia (PHE, 2016; NICE, 2015) focuses on reducing the incidence of dementia through early interventions in relation to lifestyle factors and includes alcohol reduction, exercise, smoking cessation and healthy eating, alongside mental and social stimulation.

The focus on challenging dementia at its roots by altering midlife health-related behaviours is restated in the Prime Minister's 2020 Challenge on Dementia: Implementation Plan (DHSC, 2016) and the Dementia 2020 Challenge Progress Review Part 1 (DHSC, 2019) which both recognise primary prevention as key to reducing the health-related burdens that diagnosis can place on our society. Rhys will, from this perspective, benefit from health promotion in relation to his alcohol intake, diet and exercise levels as a primary prevention-focused health promotion strategy.

David's limited social network, single status and recent retirement present 'social network' risk factors related to social isolation and loneliness, both closely associated with the onset of dementia and deterioration in mental functioning (PHE, 2016). Amieva *et al.* (2010), in a large-scale French study, identified that social support can delay the onset of dementia by up to 15 years. This reinforces the need for social contact and mental activity associated with social engagement as a means to slow the progression of the condition (Gates *et al.*, 2011; Tait *et al.*, 2017). For David health promotion would be secondary, focusing on preventing deterioration in his health status through increased social contact and mental stimulation.

For Lewis, factors relating to 'living and working' and 'general socioeconomic status' will be increasingly significant as his condition deteriorates and impacts on his functional capacity. Interventions would need to focus on financial security, his occupational security as a tenant farmer and his housing status. These factors are all associated with healthy ageing (Prince *et al.*, 2014). The focus on maintaining social and financial security and adapting to changes in functioning suggests the need for a tertiary health promotion approach concerned with maintaining activity, social functioning and daily living skills for as long as is possible.

However, it is also worth considering that primary prevention is likely to be useful for all three men. Prince *et al.* (2015) and NICE (2015) both identify that the main factors that reduce the onset and progression of cardiac conditions, vascular episodes and dementia are very similar. These include diet, exercise, mental stimulation, smoking reduction and stress management. Current research, therefore, suggests that in our present social context these common determinants present main targets for health promotion across all illness categories.

Making Every Contact Count (MECC) offers a central approach to health promotion based on this notional similarity (PHE, 2018). The aim is to focus our nursing practice on the range of common determinants of health experienced across conditions, suggesting that every time we have contact with a patient we should focus on supporting them to:

> … *improve their own lifestyle by eating well, maintaining a healthy weight, drinking alcohol sensibly, exercising regularly, not smoking and looking after their wellbeing and mental health.*

(PHE, 2018, p. 6)

This focus on improving determinants of health shifts the focus in nursing from an illness-focused approach to health promotion processes aimed at maximising health in the whole population and reducing the burden of disease at a primary, secondary and tertiary level (Prince *et al.*, 2015). MECC is focused upon further in *Chapter 6*.

### ACTIVITY 2.5

Before moving on, consider how this shift in focus, from illness to prevention and management, might affect your practice.

## 2.3 Processes that support behaviour change

### 2.3.1 Large scale approaches to changing health-related behaviours

Tannahill's model of health promotion (Tannahill, 1985; Tannahill, 2009) supports broad integrated campaigns of intervention. Tannahill challenged what he saw as an unhelpful semantic divide between health intervention, health education and health protection. Tannahill's (2009) model integrates professional intervention, health education through empowerment and legislative and social authority into one model of health promotion encouraging practitioners to use the most appropriate approach, or combination of approaches, in each situation as depicted in *Figure 2.2*.

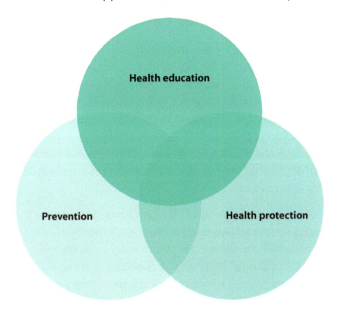

**Figure 2.2** *Tannahill's model of health promotion (adapted and simplified from materials in Tannahill, A. (1985) What is health promotion? Health Education Journal,* **44(4):** *167–8).*

National campaigns such as the Eatwell campaign (NHS England and NHS Wales) and Nutrition Skills for Life (Public Health Network Cymru, 2020) demonstrate the integration of methods of health promotion in Tannahill's (2009) model. The campaigns aim to reduce obesity by changing patterns of eating to promote sustainable health. Both campaigns use health education to inform and allow empowered decision-making. A range of multimedia education via television, visual posters and internet resources were used along with direct preventative health interventions in the form of community engagement projects and primary care screening in both campaigns and they are delivered and supported through an integration of school, NHS and broader community approaches. Legislative interventions also support change in behaviour in this area of concern and include the introduction of the MECC (PHE, 2018) process and legislation such as the introduction of the Soft Drinks Industrial Levy in 2018.

Despite such major initiatives, a recent Public Health Wales (2019) report, focusing on obesity in Wales, indicated a reduction in self-reported fruit and vegetable intake and reduced levels of healthy eating across the nation. This is contrasted in the 2019 report with an earlier data set "Welsh Health Survey" which identified a rise in health eating expenditure but no change in obesity levels in 2008. The 2019 report highlights financial barriers as a contributing factor to this increase in obesity and reduction in healthy eating. This disappointing outcome for the Eatwell campaign and the Welsh Nutrition Skills for Life initiative has led to further consideration of financial incentivisation as a mechanism to support changes in eating behaviour. This review and replanning process demonstrate the value in using well monitored national initiatives which can adapt to a changing social climate.

### 2.3.2 Theories that explain how we support change

MECC (PHE, 2018) is a major policy initiative designed to support the implementation of health promotion processes in the health and social care sector in both England and Wales. The implementation documents guide practitioners to use health promotion skills in every contact by giving information about health and wellbeing, effective relationship building, enhancing motivation in patients and supporting relevant behaviour change processes. These broad guidelines embed health promotion skills within the public service agenda for all nurse practitioners. The following section of the chapter explores some of the theories that can help us, as nurses, meet this expectation.

Michie *et al.*'s (2014) systematic review of the psychological theories that inform behavioural change identified two main categories of theory:
1. theories that explain 'how' we support change, for example medical, empowerment, educational, behavioural, cognitive and social change processes
2. theories that help us decide 'when' a specific type of intervention is most likely to succeed such as the "capacity opportunity and motivation model", the "behavioural change wheel change" and the "transtheoretical stages of change".

**Medical approaches**

Prescribed medical treatment may facilitate primary, secondary or tertiary prevention; for example, statins can be used to reduce the risk of cardiovascular disease (NICE, 2014; Rash *et al.*, 2016). However, prescribing for health is significantly problematic. While legitimated by professional expert authority, the approach rests on the assumption that the patient is willing to support this authoritative power. Let's look at an example of this notion of power in professional practice.

### ACTIVITY 2.6

Recall *Case study 2.1*; Rhys has a father with dementia and an uncle with a genetic marker and early memory loss. Today, Rhys has attended a health check at his surgery. Following the routine health screen Rhys was told that because he had a high BMI reading, he would benefit from eating a better diet and taking more exercise. It was also suggested he may need to take statins due to his high cholesterol levels. The nurse asked Rhys to follow the NHS Eatwell Guide at **www.nhs.uk/live-well/eat-well/the-eatwell-guide** and offered a follow-up in three months to review his progress.
- Is this good care?
- Are there any issues with this approach?
- Put yourself in Rhys's position. Would you feel reassured about your health, your family's health and would you eat more healthily and start to exercise?
- What was missing in this encounter?

Rhys was actually very surprised at the advice he received as he had attended the clinic because his family history had made him worry about his risk of developing dementia and he had wanted to discuss this. However, the nurse did not ask him about his needs but, instead, followed a traditional medical approach.

Despite the dominance of this approach, where the expert prescribes the actions that should be taken by the patient, it is very poor at altering behaviour. For example, reviews of the prescribing of statins identify over 50% non-compliance with the prescription (Rash *et al.*, 2016). This suggests the use of a prescription, including the Eatwell guide, may be a limited approach to health promotion.

**Empowerment**

In contrast to the encounter described in *Activity 2.6*, the MECC (PHE, 2018) guidelines suggest nurses should take an approach that enables and empowers people to change. Central to this approach is the notion of co-production and collaboration in the design and delivery of health promotion. This involves the nurse working in partnership with the patient to understand the need for change, to identify the targets for change and to select approaches to meeting these targets (PHE, 2018). This approach empowers the patient by giving them ownership and control of the process of change.

> **ACTIVITY 2.7**
>
> Returning to *Case study 2.1*, consider how this might work with Lewis, Rhys's father. Identify what you might need to do to collaborate with Lewis, who already has symptoms of dementia and is working hard to maximise his functional independence.
> - How might you integrate the familiar aspects of Lewis's life into the health-promoting activities you plan together?
> - What skills might be needed to work collaboratively and share understandings with Lewis?
> - Would you include Margaret, Lewis's wife, in the process too?
> - What might collaborative practice look like in this context?

Beattie's model of health promotion is an integrative model that allows the nurse to consider how they will approach a health need (Beattie, 1991). As demonstrated in *Figure 2.3*, Beattie presents us with a matrix of change, set on a vertical and horizontal axis. On the vertical axis the patient's behaviour is seen as influenced by the application of 'authority' at one end and 'negotiation' at the other end. On the horizontal, Beattie sets one end as individual action and the other as collective or social action. Expert practitioners use individual authority or persuasion to gain compliance but may also use collective legal or socially endorsed processes to ensure compliance. At the authority end of the continuum we are considering compliance rather than collaboration or concordance.

## Chapter 2: Behaviour change: theories, models and approaches

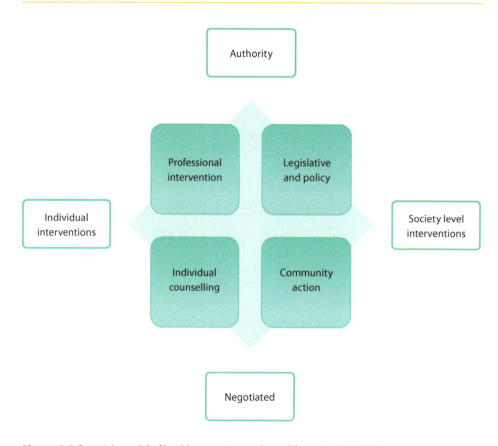

**Figure 2.3** *Beattie's model of health promotion, adapted from Beattie (1991).*

Beattie's (1991) model reminds us that health promotion is complex and as nurses we are in a position where we must decide ethically about the different approaches that are most appropriate to meet the patient's needs in their particular context. The following case study allows us to explore this in relation to James, who has type 1 diabetes.

> **CASE STUDY 2.2A  JAMES**
>
> James presents at the Emergency Department (ED) of your hospital. He is agitated, confused and aggressive. He appears incoherent and shows you his medic alert bracelet. He has been in the ED previously and is well known to the nurse manager. He has type 1 diabetes which is poorly controlled. You watch the nurse manager intervene. They begin by using a rational imperative, insisting that James sits down. James complies with this. They then take a blood sugar reading. James is hypoglycaemic.
>
> As James recovers, he appears tearful and remorseful. The nurse manager tells him about healthy eating and leaves him with the NHS Eatwell weblink. James says he only wants to be normal again, like he used to be.

## ACTIVITY 2.8

Consider *Case study 2.2a*:
- What kind of relationship was the nurse using here?
- Was this appropriate?
- What health promotion approach was in operation?
- What is the likely outcome of the nurse's intervention?
- Consider other health promotion options available for James.
- Which of Beattie's four paradigms are most appropriate?

You probably recognise that the nurse was using an expert position, using professional authority to ensure James complied with treatment. This was an authoritative approach to James's health needs. The treatment was a prescribed treatment and the approach was not collaborative or negotiated. If the nurse had used Beattie's matrix and selected a negotiated approach this may have enhanced the intervention, allowing the patient to share decision-making and ownership of their own behaviour. In this context the patient became a passive recipient of care. Beattie's model is helpful in that it encourages us to consider and select levers of change that empower and support behavioural change in each context. While authoritative practice has its place in emergency treatment, a shared decision-making approach, which Beattie would call counselling, may have offered a better way forward for James.

**Health education programmes**

Sharing information with our patients creates a capacity for people to self-manage their care and to make appropriate decisions about their health.

The Dose Adjustment For Normal Eating (DAFNE) educational programme educates adults with type 1 diabetes to manage their insulin, diet and exercise. The programme is delivered through a five-day intensive course run across the country by trained providers (Diabetes UK, 2019). DAFNE offers a bespoke and personalised approach to training using peer groups and professional input alongside psychoeducation to provide motivation and support for change. Reviews of the DAFNE programme indicate clinical benefit in key indicators including QOL and HbA1c levels (Heller *et al.*, 2014). This programme would have been useful for James to help him manage his diabetes and the challenges of regular insulin therapy.

BERTIE (Beta Cell Education Resources for Training in Insulin and Eating) would offer a similar resource for James. The programme was initially developed as an alternative to DAFNE as a 4-day group training programme focused on problem solving and education. BERTIE online also offers an alternative delivery mode which is more accessible. Modular learning experiences are accessed through the website www.bertieonline.org.uk. The BERTIE project, developed by the Bournemouth Diabetes and Endocrine Department, provides open access resources allowing tailored problem-solving for each patient.

The above examples of education for people with type 1 diabetes both demonstrate that a well designed health education intervention requires more than the delivery of facts. Both DAFNE and BERTIE use individualised tailoring of response and peer and professional support to solve and resolve real-life problems around behavioural change. Nurses delivering health education need to take into account the information needed by their patients and help them select the most useful materials from networked resources, such as the DAFNE and BERTIE programmes, to resolve their bespoke barriers to change.

> **ACTIVITY 2.9**
>
> In *Case study 2.2a*, James's nurse assumed that supplying James with the internet link would provide sufficient information for him to change his behaviour.
> - Consider the NHS Eatwell campaign information: bit.ly/2-9A
> - How does this alternative information compare?: bit.ly/2-9B
> - What do you notice about the quality, digestibility and accessibility of the information presented in these two resources?

Effective health education provides information that is relevant to the patient, accessible and easily digestible. When designed well and used sensitively to reflect the patient's needs and context it can inform evidence-based decision-making (Naidoo and Wills, 2016). The well-known Australian programme to reduce skin cancer which began as the "slip, slop, slap" campaign in 1980 was a significant piece of health education. This early campaign was primarily a TV campaign along with other advertising processes to deliver a clear message in three parts: Slip on a T-shirt, Slop on sun protection lotion and Slap on a hat. The campaign continued for 8 years until it was replaced with the SunSmart campaign (Montague, Borland and Sinclair, 2001). The clear use of the mnemonic to remind people to slip, slop and slap, alongside education on the health burden and benefits of this behaviour, led to significant change in behaviour at a population level. The SunSmart programme used a more integrated pattern of community engagement through school, health centre and community initiatives to increase protective behaviours to reduce skin cancer, thereby extending the existing slip, slop, slap programme. Over a period of 40 years the incidence of early skin cancer in the population has dropped by approximately 5% each year (Montague, Borland and Sinclair, 2001; Tabbakh *et al.*, 2019).

However, caution is needed, because despite the global benefit of large scale health promotion approaches such as the SunSmart programme and the less compelling effectiveness of the Eatwell programme, the literature suggests that these approaches do not effectively target those most at risk at the individual level and they can have a low level of uptake (Sinclair and Foley, 2009).

Targeting at-risk individuals like James and personalising the information-giving process may be necessary if we are to change health-related behaviours in at-risk individuals. The remaining components of the chapter focus on this notion of personalised and targeted health promotion with individuals.

### ACTIVITY 2.10

Consider how you could personalise the health education given to James (*Case study 2.2a*) to help him understand and act upon the material presented to him by the nurse. Make some notes before moving on.

## 2.4 Overcoming barriers to change

Smaller scale behavioural change requires a different level of understanding to that outlined above. Michie *et al.* (2014) systematically reviewed the amassing body of research focusing on how people change their behaviours. The ABC of behaviour change (Michie *et al.*, 2014) is a compendium of behavioural change theories that can inform our practice when working with patients to support their efforts to change, and offers an excellent resource for those wishing to extend their knowledge.

Within this chapter we will consider just two of the psychological models that were developed to help us understand how people change their behaviour. The initial model, "the theory of reasoned action" will be discussed first. This is a seminal model and is the bedrock for many of the more recent theories. The second approach will be the most recent model developed by Michie *et al.* (2014) from the systematic review of psychological theories. The "behaviour change wheel" provides an integration of the knowledge and practice models currently used. As we explore the two models, we will focus on how nurses can use this type of theory to enhance their work with patients.

### 2.4.1 The theory of reasoned action

The theory of reasoned action was first published in 1967 by Fishbein and then reviewed by Ajzen and Fishbein (1980) and Ajzen and Albarracin (2007). It is one of the earliest theories developed to help us understand how people move from health education to behavioural change. The theory assumes that people use rational decision-making to underpin reasoned action. Recently theorists have challenged the rational position, suggesting impulsive action and emotional decision-making may also be important (Michie, van Stralen and West, 2011). For now, we will consider what this theory has to offer. The theory focuses on building intention to act. Intention is influenced by previous learning including beliefs about change, other beliefs about a new behaviour, attitudes towards change and our intention to change. All the factors mediate between knowledge and action and, therefore, either ease or present barriers to change. The theory has relevance to nurses as we work to reduce these barriers and enhance the levers for change. *Figure 2.4* identifies these component elements of the model.

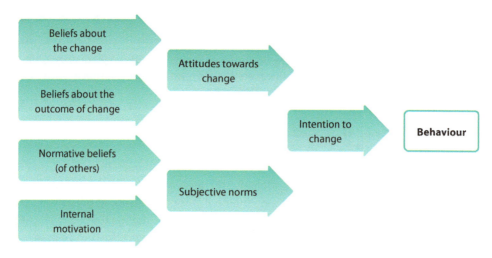

**Figure 2.4** The components of the theory of reasoned action (adapted from the original by Ajzen and Fishbein, 1980).

To get a better understanding of the application of this model let's apply Ajzen and Fishbein's theory to James, whom we met earlier.

### CASE STUDY 2.2B JAMES

James has begun to explore with his nurse the need to change his approach to food and is keen to stay well for as long as possible. He states that he believes that this will be good for him (outcome-focused beliefs) but that he *"will never be able to eat properly"* and *"even if I did it still wouldn't be enough to control my blood glucose"* (evaluation of outcome). His attitude to change his behaviour to eat a balanced diet is clearly ambivalent, which he summarises in the statement *"I know I should eat differently to stay well, but I don't see how it is going to help me to get better"* (attitude). James's intention to begin to eat a balanced diet is limited by this attitude which he states as *"I can't do it at the moment as it will not work for me"* (intention). James, therefore, continues to binge and then starve, further exacerbating the fluctuations in blood sugar he experiences.

However, James is also influenced by his family, friends and his specialist nurse (normative beliefs) who tell him that balanced eating will be good for him. He particularly wants to please his nurse, which increases his motivation to change (internal motivation). James's attitude to balancing his eating derived from others (subjective norms) influences James to identify eating a balanced diet as a valued change in behaviour.

James is torn between acting in accordance with his own attitude to change and his evaluation of the outcome and those of the people around him.

After James's specialist nurse explores his understanding of the relationship between a balanced diet and stabilising his blood glucose levels with him (normative beliefs), James re-evaluates his own beliefs and attitudes towards the change (attitude) and becomes excited about feeling healthier. James and his specialist nurse spend some time building a realistic plan for balanced eating and this begins to build his intent to act (intent).

James is now eating well and has not been to the emergency department for 3 months. The risk to his eyesight and peripheral nervous system are now significantly lower. James's blood glucose levels are stabilising and he has been told by his GP that he may be able to reduce the frequency of his insulin injections.

## 2.4 Overcoming barriers to change

The case study highlights that by carefully examining outcome-focused beliefs, evaluative beliefs and attitudes to change with our patients, we can begin to see what is impacting on their ability to change and this will increase their intent to act. Did you notice that intent was also enhanced by joint planning of specific, measurable, achievable, realistic and time-bound (SMART) goals for action (PHE, 2018)?

While not designed specifically for this purpose, using this kind of model begins to help patients understand the barriers to change they are experiencing and to address these so that change can occur.

### 2.4.2 Pender's health promotion model

Pender's health promotion model (Pender, 1982) focuses attention on barriers to change similar to those we examined above. Pender emphasises the motivational barriers to change and the value of the relationship we develop with our patients during nursing practice. Pender suggests we can mobilise our relationship to help patients build homeostasis by supporting health-enhancing patterns of thinking and doing. James's case above clearly highlights Pender's approach, where the nursing relationship is used to enhance the patient's motivation to change. The model focuses on concepts such as motivation and self-esteem as mediators of change and it highlights a need to use the nursing relationship to build the patient's self-belief and motivation. This use of our relationship to model and support change is termed "the social cognitive approach". Pender builds her model around this social cognitive position, using our nursing influence to empower and guide the patient towards and through sometimes difficult change.

> **ACTIVITY 2.11**
>
> Consider the subjective and personal assumptions and beliefs that might be barriers to a patient's change process. Consider how as a nurse you empower the patient and help them to overcome doubt and believe in the change process. You may want to consider a situation in which the patient wishes to stop smoking but their friends and family all smoke. What would you need to do to model and demonstrate a new normative position to the patient? How could you enable and support their internal motivation and external intention to change?

### 2.4.3 COM B

The "Capacity Opportunity and Motivation = Behaviour (COM-B)" model (Michie, van Stralen and West, 2011; Michie *et al.*, 2014) offers an overarching model of change that helps us identify clearly the potential barriers to change that a patient is experiencing and helps us target our intervention effectively. It provides a simple integration of three areas for intervention to maximise change. These areas are capacity, opportunity and motivation (COM) which, when addressed, lead to behavioural change (B). This model is recommended in the MECC (PHE, 2018) guidance to support interventions.

Capacity is the ability to do the task and might include the skills and knowledge necessary to undertake the task, as well as the underlying intellectual or behavioural ability. In James's case (*Case studies 2.2a* and *2.2b*) he may have capacity issues concerning insufficient knowledge and skills to be able to prepare food and this may become a central target in order to promote change in his diet.

Opportunity includes the resources the person might have to support the change in behaviour. This might be social resources, including supportive others and access to networks of support, as well as physical resources, including access to environments or equipment as well as finance and travel. If James is concerned that his friends may not understand that he requires food regularly and that alcohol is likely to cause fluctuations in his blood glucose levels, a second focus for intervention to support behavioural change may include educating his friends or helping James engage in a more supportive and progressive social network.

Motivation relates to the person's willingness to engage in the behaviour. This will be affected by their beliefs about the behaviour, its value, their perceptions regarding their ability to undertake the required action and whether it is a priority for them at that point in time.

### ACTIVITY 2.12

As practitioners, these three areas (COM) can be incorporated into a plan for change. Consider the COM-B model for one of your own patients by completing the table below.

|  | Capacity | Opportunity | Motivation |
|---|---|---|---|
| Deficits or areas to address |  |  |  |
| Intervention needed to overcome deficits |  |  |  |
| Intervention to build on opportunities |  |  |  |

The COM-B model allows you to work with your patients to overcome barriers to change. You may want to use this kind of table in practice to support the change process in action. Take some time to consider the table and how it would help you identify interventions based on your relationship with the patient or social cognitive influences.

## 2.4.4 Behavioural change wheel

Working alongside the COM-B model, Michie, van Stralen and West (2011) developed the behavioural change wheel. The behavioural change wheel represents a synthesis model, much like Dahlgren and Whitehead's (1991) earlier determinant-based model, creating an integrated theory to support clinical decision-making in relation to what works for whom. The model includes three interacting rings; the first, at a personal level, identifies the barrier to change in each situation using the COM-B tool above. The second ring identifies the main intervention techniques and approaches available to promote change and the third ring (the outer rim) identifies a range of authoritative social levers that can be applied to legitimate enforced change. When you examine the model (*Figure 2.5*) you will note many similarities with Beattie's (1991) model, which also includes authoritative and negotiated elements and directs the reader to differentiate between individual and broader social mechanisms for change.

### ACTIVITY 2.13

Consider how the behavioural change wheel might offer you a method to select and use a broader range of health promotion processes in your practice. As you examine the wheel, consider what value it has to you as a nurse and what limitations it may have.

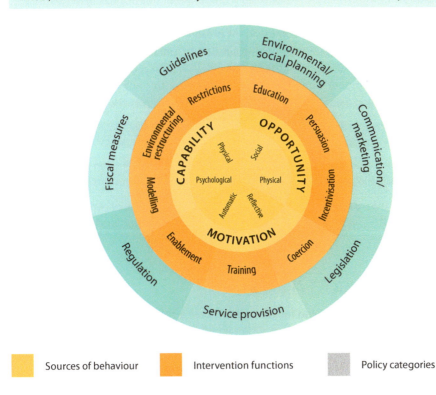

**Figure 2.5** *The behaviour change wheel. Reproduced with permission from Michie, S., Atkins, L. and West, R. (2014)* The Behaviour Change Wheel: a guide to designing interventions. *London: Silverback Publishing. www.behaviourchangewheel.com*

### ACTIVITY 2.14

Read Michie, van Stralen and West's (2011) article, Michie *et al.*'s (2014) taxonomised compendium of behavioural change theories and visit this website to find out more about this innovative tool: www.bct-taxonomy.com

As you explore, keep in mind the unique relationship you have with patients and how this can be used to help patients clarify their understandings and goals.

## 2.5 Building motivation to change

Motivational interviewing offers an evidence-based approach to overcoming barriers to change. It is a directive, patient-focused approach that uses a range of approaches focused on listening and questioning to enhance change-oriented self-talk (Miller and Rollnick, 2012). The main processes are rolling with resistance, exploring discrepancies between actual and desired behaviours and using change-focused questioning. The RCN (2019) supports the use of this approach in health promotion practice and has developed training tools to build the capacity of the workforce in delivering health promotion. At present motivational interviewing offers the most tested form of talking intervention to initiate and sustain changes in behaviour, and any nursing practitioner who sees health promotion as a central component of their practice needs to seriously consider this approach within their toolkit. A further discussion of motivational interviewing is provided in *Chapter 6*.

### ACTIVITY 2.15

Motivational interviewing is deceptively simple in design but difficult to do in practice. Watch these RCN clips and identify which would be most useful for you: bit.ly/2-15A

To understand the core skills in full, the five Australian Heart Foundation videos at the following link offer you an excellent starting point to develop motivational skills: bit.ly/2-15B

## 2.6 Setting a plan for change

Goal setting and building a plan for change requires a collaborative approach to identify SMART plans. This process, when conducted effectively, can be self-motivating for patients since it gives them control of the intervention and provides regular opportunities to succeed.

## 2.6 Setting a plan for change

> **ACTIVITY 2.16**
>
> When planning behavioural changes with James to target balanced eating and blood glucose regulation, what kind of approach would you take? What relationship would you foster with James? Who would write the plan down? What kind of short-, medium- and long-term goals might you set with James?

In undertaking *Activity 2.16* you may have considered how together you might break up the tasks set for the short-term goal, to allow James to experience self-reinforcing success right from the outset. You may have also considered the measurable elements of the process and how often blood glucose levels and HbA1c may be measured to reinforce the health gains. While improved HbA1c will be a priority for you as a healthcare professional, for James the more immediate changes in his blood glucose levels and his general sense of wellbeing may be of greater relevance.

At this point in the book, you should have started to develop a set of skills that can help manage change-focused relationships, empower change through shared understanding and informed decision-making and support change focused towards enhancing health. The final strand to behavioural change theory considers the timing of interventions.

### 2.6.1 The stages of change model

The stages of change model (Prochaska and DiClemente, 1986) originated in the field of substance misuse counselling, but has been widely used across a range of public health and health promotion initiatives since its inception. It is transtheoretical, making an assumption that all people who are changing will travel through a similar set of stages regardless of the change they are making. *Figure 2.6* outlines the movement between the six stages of change, which are:

- Pre-contemplative: focuses on helping the individual recognise that a need to change exists
- Contemplative: focuses on helping the individual consider whether they are ready to change
- Preparation: concerned with change-orientated planning aimed at helping the individual consider how they might change
- Action: implementation of behaviour change
- Maintenance: focuses on helping the individual maintain new behaviour by rewarding changed behaviour
- Termination: either achieved when lifestyle change has been permanently achieved or focuses on helping the individual examine and learn from periods of relapse.

*Chapter 2: Behaviour change: theories, models and approaches*

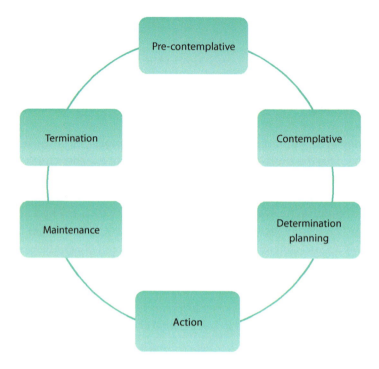

**Figure 2.6** *The stages of change model (adapted from Prochaska and DiClemente (1986)).*

### ACTIVITY 2.17

The stages of change model focuses attention on the specific stage in the change process related to the patient's needs. Consider the following intervention made by a practice nurse supporting James (*Case studies 2.2a* and *2.2b*). What stage of change is James at and what options for intervention are there for him at each stage?

- James was discharged from the ED and has now stabilised, but he has a very high HbA1c of 119mmol/mol and the GP is concerned about his physical health. James is seen for a routine check-up and states he doesn't see a problem with his HbA1c – it has been like that for a while and doesn't bother him at all.
- After two more visits James accepts that his HbA1c is worrying, but he is unsure if he is ready to do anything about it.
- After a further two visits James states he needs to do something about his health but he doesn't know how to go about it and feels he doesn't have the capability to change.
- After a further period of a month James has begun a diabetes management programme and is using a fitness app. He comes to you stating he feels it is taking too long to notice any change and is disappointed.
- After a further two weeks of the programme James has begun to feel more in control of his diet and his blood sugars are now regulated, with no more dizziness or fainting. However, he confides he had some chocolate last week and ate the whole bar.
- After a further three months of the programme James's HbA1c has reduced and he has joined an organisation working in the local mental health hospital to support patients to gain control of their diabetes.

While thinking about the stages of change, you may have matched James's needs with educational approaches, empowerment, behavioural planning and discussions regarding beliefs and attitudes towards change, depending upon his needs at each stage of behavioural change. Process theories, like the stages of change model, allow you to see what needs to be done at what point to help the individual move through a journey of change. A further example of how the stages of change model can be applied in practice is provided in *Chapter 6*.

> **KEY LEARNING POINTS**
>
> Five key points to take away from *Chapter 2*:
> - Behavioural change theory helps us, as nurses, to understand how people make changes in their behaviours, and which behaviours can provide effective gains in health.
> - Clinical guidelines through programmes such as Making Every Contact Count focus our attention on the range of activities that support health promotion.
> - A variety of health promotion and behavioural change models can be applied to help us empower patients to change.
> - Collaborative exploration, goal setting and behavioural planning, recognising and planning to overcome barriers to change and promoting progress towards a change orientation all offer effective mechanisms a nurse can use to support change.
> - The nurse is in a unique and powerful position as an agent of change.

# REFERENCES

Ajzen, I. and Albarracin, D. (2007) 'Predicting and changing behaviour: a reasoned action approach'. In Ajzen, I., Albarracin, D. and Hornik, R. (eds) *Prediction and Change of Health Behavior: applying the reasoned action approach*. Lawrence Erlbaum Associates.

Ajzen, I. and Fishbein, M. (1980) *Understanding Attitudes and Predicting Social Behavior*. Prentice-Hall.

Alzheimer's Research UK (2018) *Prevalence*. Available at: www.dementiastatistics.org/statistics-about-dementia/prevalence (accessed 7 May 2020)

Amieva, H., Stoykova, R., Matharan, F. *et al.* (2010) What aspects of social network are protective for dementia? Not the quantity but the quality of social interactions is protective up to 15 years later. *Psychosomatic Medicine*, **72(9)**: 905–11.

Beattie, A. (1991) 'Knowledge and control in health promotion: a test case for social policy and theory'. In Gabe, J., Calnan, M. and Bury, M. (eds) *The Sociology of the Health Service*. Taylor and Francis.

Cragg, L., Davies, M. and MacDowall, W. (2013) *Health Promotion Theory*, 2nd edition. Open University Press.

Dahlgren, G. and Whitehead, M. (1991) *Policies and Strategies to Promote Social Equity in Health*. Stockholm Institute for Futures Studies.

Department of Health and Social Care (2016) *Prime Minister's Challenge on Dementia 2020 Implementation Plan*. Available at: https://assets.publishing.service.gov.uk/government/uploads/system/uploads/attachment_data/file/507981/PM_Dementia-main_acc.pdf (accessed 7 May 2020)

Department of Health and Social Care (2019) *Dementia 2020 Challenge: 2018 Review Phase 1*. Available at: https://assets.publishing.service.gov.uk/government/uploads/system/uploads/attachment_data/file/780777/dementia-2020-challenge-2018-review.pdf (accessed 7 May 2020)

Diabetes UK (2019) DAFNE – Dose Adjustment for Normal Eating. Available at: www.diabetes.co.uk/education/dafne.html (accessed 7 July 2020)

Gates, N., Sachdev, P., Fiatarone Singh, M. and Valenzuela, M. (2011) Cognitive and memory training in adults at risk of dementia: a systematic review. *BMC Geriatrics*, **11(55)**: (2011) doi:10.1186/1471-2318-11-55.

Heginbotham, C. and Newbigging, K. (2013) *Commissioning Health and Wellbeing*. SAGE.

Heller, S., Lawton, J., Amiel, S. *et al.* (2014) Improving management of type 1 diabetes in the UK: the Dose Adjustment For Normal Eating (DAFNE) programme as a research test-bed. A mixed-method analysis of the barriers to and facilitators of successful diabetes self-management, a health economic analysis, a cluster randomised controlled trial of different models of delivery of an educational intervention and the potential of insulin pumps and additional educator input to improve outcomes. *Programme Grants for Applied Research*, No. 2.5. Available at: www.ncbi.nlm.nih.gov/books/NBK263961/ (accessed 7 May 2020)

Marmot, M. (2010) *Fair Society, Healthy Lives*. Available at: www.parliament.uk/documents/fair-society-healthy-lives-full-report.pdf (accessed 6 May 2020)

Marmot, M. (2020) *Health Equity in England: the Marmot review 10 years on*. Institute of Health Equity. Available at: www.health.org.uk/sites/default/files/upload/publications/2020/Health%20Equity%20in%20England_The%20Marmot%20Review%2010%20Years%20On_full%20report.pdf (accessed 6 May 2020)

Michie, S., van Stralen, M. and West, R. (2011) The behaviour change wheel: a new method for characterising and designing behaviour change interventions. *Implementation Science*, **6(42)**: doi:10.1186/1748-5908-6-42.

Michie S., Atkins L. and West, R. (2014) *The Behaviour Change Wheel: a guide to designing interventions*. Silverback Publishing. www.behaviourchangewheel.com

Michie, S., West, R., Campbell, R., Brown, J. and Gainforth, H. (2014) *ABC of Behaviour Change Theories: an essential resource for researchers, policy makers and practitioners*. Silverback Publishing.

Miller, W. and Rollnick, S. (2012) *Motivational Interviewing: helping people change*. Guilford Press.

Montague, M., Borland, R. and Sinclair, C. (2001) Slip! Slop! Slap! and SunSmart, 1980–2000: skin cancer control and 20 years of population-based campaigning. *Health Education and Behaviour*, **28(3):** 290–305.

Murdaugh, C., Parsons, M. and Pender, N. (2019) *Health Promotion in Nursing Practice*, 8th edition. Pearson Publishing.

Naidoo, J. and Wills, J. (2016) *Foundations for Health Promotion*, 4th edition. Elsevier.

NICE (2014) CG181 *Cardiovascular disease: risk assessment and reduction, including lipid modification*. Available at: www.nice.org.uk/guidance/CG181 (accessed 7 May 2020)

NICE (2015) NG16 *Dementia, disability and frailty in later life – mid-life approaches to delay or prevent onset*. Available at: www.nice.org.uk/guidance/ng16 (accessed 7 May 2020)

Norton, S. Matthews, F., Barnes, D., Yaffe, K. and Brayne, C. (2014) Potential for primary prevention of Alzheimer's disease: an analysis of population-based data. *The Lancet Neurology*, **13(8):** 788–94.

Pender, N. (1982) *Health Promotion in Nursing Practice*. Appleton-Century-Crofts.

Prince, M., Knapp, M., Guerchet, M. *et al*. (2014) *Dementia UK*, 2nd edition. Available at: http://eprints.lse.ac.uk/59437/1/Dementia_UK_Second_edition_-_Overview.pdf (accessed 7 May 2020)

Prince, M., Wu, F., Guo, Y. *et al*. (2015) The burden of disease in older people and implications for health policy and practice. *Lancet*, **385(9967):** 549–62.

Prochaska, J. and DiClemente, C. (1986) 'Toward a comprehensive model of change'. In Miller, W. and Heather, N. (eds) *Treating Addictive Behaviors: processes of change*. Plenum Press.

Public Health England (2016) *Health Matters: midlife approaches to reduce dementia risk*. Available at: www.gov.uk/government/publications/health-matters-midlife-approaches-to-reduce-dementia-risk/health-matters-midlife-approaches-to-reduce-dementia-risk (accessed 7 May 2020)

Public Health England (2018) *Making Every Contact Count (MECC): implementation guide*. Available at: https://assets.publishing.service.gov.uk/government/uploads/system/uploads/attachment_data/file/769488/MECC_Implememenation_guide_v2.pdf (accessed 7 May 2020)

Public Health Network Cymru (2020) *Making Every Contact Count (MECC): web resources*. Available at: https://mecc.publichealthnetwork.cymru/en/resources (accessed 7 May 2020)

Public Health Wales (2019) *Obesity in Wales*. Available at: www.publichealthwalesobservatory.wales.nhs.uk/sitesplus/documents/1208/ObesityInWales_Report2018_v1.pdf (accessed 7 May 2020)

Rash, J., Campbell, D., Tonelli, M. and Campbell, T. (2016) A systematic review of interventions to improve adherence to statin medication: what do we know about what works? *Preventative Medicine*, **90**: 155–69.

Royal College of Nursing (2019) *Supporting Behaviour Change*. Available at: www.rcn.org.uk/clinical-topics/supporting-behaviour-change (accessed 7 May 2020)

Sinclair, C. and Foley, P. (2009) Skin cancer prevention in Australia. *British Journal of Dermatology*, **161:** 116–23.

Tabbakh, T., Volkov, A., Wakefield, M., and Dobbinson, S. (2019) Implementation of the SunSmart program and population sun protection behaviour in Melbourne, Australia: results from cross-sectional summer surveys from 1987 to 2017. PLoS Med, **16(10):** e1002932. Available at: https://doi.org/10.1371/journal.pmed.1002932 (accessed 7 May 2020)

Tait, J., Duckham, R., Milte, C., Main, L. and Daly, R. (2017) Influence of sequential vs. simultaneous dual-task exercise training on cognitive functioning in older adults. *Frontiers in Aging Neuroscience*, **9(368):** doi.org/10.3389/fnagi.2017.00368.

Tannahill, A. (1985) What is health promotion? *Health Education Journal,* **44(4):** 167–8.

Tannahill, A. (2009) Health promotion: the Tannahill model revisited. *Public Health*, **123(5):** 396–9.

# Chapter 3
# Inequalities in health

Beverley Johnson

> **LEARNING OUTCOMES**
>
> When you have finished this chapter, you should be able to:
>
> **3.1** Define inequalities in health
>
> **3.2** Identify the social determinants of health that affect a person throughout the life course
>
> **3.3** Outline key studies regarding health inequalities
>
> **3.4** List the social and economic influences on gender and health
>
> **3.5** List the social and economic influences on ethnicity and health.

## 3.1 Introduction

Unless you have studied sociology previously you may not realise that inequalities in health are a major problem for the UK and that this has real relevance for nurses. This chapter will highlight that ill health is unevenly weighted, with the poorest in society carrying the greatest burden.

There are some groups in the UK that are more likely to die early and to have worse health. The fact that different groups experience different levels of health is known as inequalities in health. These health differences are often measured using mortality rates, disability and life expectancy at birth. There are differences in health and ill health between the UK and other countries in the world, between different areas of the UK and between different social groups. For example, lung cancer is more prevalent amongst the most deprived groups in society (Sanderson *et al.*, 2018).

Some health inequalities, such as breast cancer, are the result of biological differences between sexes and others between different races, such as sickle cell anaemia. However, the term largely relates to unfair, systemic differences in health outcomes between groups that are avoidable (King's Fund, 2020).

Inequalities in health concern differences in life expectancy at birth, mortality and morbidity. There is a social gradient in lifespan in the UK; people living in the most deprived areas of the UK can expect to live up to ten years less than those in the least deprived areas. Furthermore, they can expect to spend twenty years in worse health, spending nearly a third of their lives in poor health (PHE, 2017a). In comparison, those in the least deprived areas can expect to live in poor health for only a sixth of their lives. Nearly half of the gap in life expectancy between the most and least deprived areas of the UK is related to excess deaths from heart disease, stroke and cancer (PHE, 2017a). These differences in health outcomes are underpinned by inequalities in the social and economic circumstances which influence health. The causes of these inequalities are known as social determinants of health.

This chapter will identify patterns in inequalities in health and identify those most disadvantaged in society and susceptible to poor health; it will then explore some of the social determinants of health. This is particularly relevant for nurses when providing health promotion, as nurses need to understand the challenges that some people are faced with when making choices about their health. We cannot assume that people have the resources to make healthy changes.

## 3.2 The history of health inequalities

You will come across a number of different terms in this chapter. Some common terms and their definitions are:

- **Life expectancy at birth**: this is the average number of years that a newborn is expected to live if current mortality rates continue to apply (WHO, 2006)
- **Mortality**: this relates to death (Hernandez and Kim, 2020)
- **Morbidity**: refers to being unhealthy from a disease or condition (Hernandez and Kim, 2020).

Significant differences in life expectancy at birth, mortality and morbidity have been found in different groups in society. For example, differences in health outcomes vary according to social class, gender and ethnicity. Researchers have found that the greater the person's socioeconomic position, the better their health and vice versa (Townsend, Davidson and Whitehead, 1988). Since the early part of the twentieth century, inequalities in health have been measured by social class based on occupation. This was a very crude measure and was fraught with difficulties. Women were classified according to their husband's occupation and, as occupation was a very heterogeneous concept, it was not necessarily indicative of income or behaviour.

More recently, research has moved away from this type of measure to focus instead on areas of deprivation using the indices of deprivation. These allow the individual countries of the UK to examine geographical areas and the multiple factors that contribute to relative deprivation. Each country measures deprivation slightly differently; however, they all include income, employment, health, education, access to services, housing, community safety and physical environment. Areas of greatest deprivation have less access to those resources.

## ACTIVITY 3.1

For each of the measures outlined above, make a list of how you think they can influence health.

What is the nurse's role in addressing these factors?

As you will see in *Chapter 5*, nurses can have an impact upon all of these factors through mediating, enabling and advocating with and for patients and populations.

In order to understand inequalities in health it is helpful to know the key studies that have been published in the last 40 years:

The Black Report (Townsend, Davidson and Whitehead, 1988) is the seminal piece of work that demonstrated that health is not evenly distributed within society. The Black Report clearly identified that health was influenced by social class and those in the lower classes were more likely to die early and have worse health. The Black Report presented four possible explanations for inequalities in health:

*Artefact:* this suggested that the evidence on inequalities in health was due to the measuring processes and that inequalities may not be as prevalent as they appeared. However, through a thorough analysis of the evidence, the Black Report concluded that this was not a plausible explanation and inequalities in health existed.

*Social selection:* this theory suggests that people in the worst health will be more prone to poverty due to poor education and occupation. The evidence explored in the Black Report identified that this theory was rather weak in explaining health inequalities.

*Behavioural/cultural:* this theory suggests that those who are in the most deprived areas are more likely to have poor health-related behaviour, such as smoking and a poor diet. There is some evidence to support this theory, but the Black Report favoured the materialistic explanation.

*Materialistic:* the report concluded that material circumstances had the greatest impact on health. They specifically identified income, housing, education, employment and conditions of work as having a direct effect on health and ill health and an indirect effect on health-related behaviours. The report recommended that social policy should focus on reducing social inequalities. However, the report was ignored by the government at that time. Public health measures have subsequently largely focused on addressing the behavioural aspects of health, such as diet and smoking, through health promotion and health education measures.

Since the publication of the Black Report, a breadth of evidence has accumulated analysing social and economic factors as determinants of health, and there has been an increase in prospective and longitudinal studies which study people over a period of time. For example, the Whitehall study (Marmot *et al.*, 1991, 1997), which is a longitudinal study of British civil servants, found inequalities in health and mortality between employment grades. It found that risk factors such as being overweight, having high levels of cholesterol and smoking could only explain one-third of the differences in health by employment grade. The study concluded that much of the difference in health status can be explained by work autonomy and control.

The Acheson Report (1988), which provided an independent inquiry into health inequalities, found that mortality had decreased in the last 50 years but that inequalities in health remained and, in some instances, had worsened. The report identified a very complex interplay of factors. The aim of the paper was to inform and advise the government on public health policy and it made the following recommendations:

- Health impact assessments should be implemented for all policies that are likely to have a direct or indirect impact on health and health inequalities.
- High priority should be given to the health of families with children.
- Further steps should be taken to reduce income inequalities and improve the living standards of poor households.

Thirty years on, the Marmot Review (Marmot, 2010) published *Fair Society, Healthy Lives*, a review into inequalities in health. The results showed that inequalities in health persist in the UK. People in the poorest areas of England were predicted to die seven years earlier than those in the richest areas and spend approximately seventeen years in worse health. Marmot (2010) also showed that the causes were a combination of income, housing, education and social isolation and cost the UK about £40 billion.

More recently, the Institute of Health Equity (2018) has found that in the ten years since the publication of the Marmot Review, health inequalities appear to be widening, with death and morbidity more prevalent in the disadvantaged groups. In 2020 Marmot published *Health Equity in England: the Marmot review 10 years on*, which demonstrated a further widening of health inequalities. The review identified that inequalities in life expectancy have increased further, particularly for women, and regional inequalities in life expectancy have also increased, with life expectancy lower in the north and higher in the south. Inequalities in health, therefore, persist as a major public health challenge in the 21st century.

### ACTIVITY 3.2

The publications above have identified several social determinants of health such as housing, education and income. Make a list of questions to ask your patients that might identify some of the social factors which may contribute to their health status. Next, list members of the multidisciplinary teams that nurses work with, who may be important in supporting patients from areas of deprivation.

## 3.3 Statistical evidence

This part of the chapter will summarise national data which serves as a barometer of the social and economic conditions in which people live. As mentioned in *Section 3.2*, deprivation is measured using indices of deprivation.

The report from the Office for National Statistics (ONS, 2019) on life expectancy between 2015 and 2017 identified that in England the gap in life expectancy at birth between the least deprived and the most deprived areas was 9.4 years for males. Life expectancy for men living in the most deprived areas in England was 74 years, compared to 83 years in the least deprived areas. Life expectancy for females in the most deprived areas was 78.8 years, while females in the least deprived areas could expect to live to 86.2 years; a difference of 7.4 years.

In addition to living fewer years, both males and females can expect to live more years in poorer health if they live in a deprived area. In England healthy life expectancy for men in deprived areas is 51.7 years, compared to 70.4 years in the least deprived areas. That means that men who reside in more deprived areas can expect to live nearly 20 years in poorer health than those who are least deprived. Similarly, women in the most deprived areas could expect to live 52 years in good health, compared to 70.4 years in the least deprived areas, which again is nearly 20 years' difference (ONS, 2019).

Marmot's (2020) review outlines similar findings and emphasises that significant socioeconomic gradients explain much of this preventable morbidity and mortality. The poorest geographical areas experience greatest preventable mortality and morbidity rates and the richest areas have the least.

### ACTIVITY 3.3

Why does living in a deprived area impact so significantly upon people's health? List four reasons.

## 3.4 Explaining inequalities in health

This part of the chapter explores the relationship between social disadvantage and poor health. It will explore five different models of health inequalities identified by Bartley (2017). These include the cultural-behavioural model, the materialist model, the psychosocial model and the Spirit Level, and the life-course model.

### 3.4.1 Cultural-behavioural model

The *cultural-behavioural* approach asserts that culture determines behavioural and health choices, such as drinking, smoking or an unhealthy diet. This approach suggests that unhealthy behaviours are related to deprivation, with a greater proportion of individuals in deprived areas adopting unhealthy lifestyles (Stait and Calnan, 2016). However, this tells us little of the context in which these behaviours occur, or how they are influenced by the social and economic environment. It is important that we do not portray individuals as victims of their own ignorance. Traditionally it was believed that there was a lack of knowledge in the lower social groups concerning the potential harm of certain behaviours, such as smoking or drinking excess alcohol and health promotion activities have been targeted at improving individuals' knowledge. However, very few people are ignorant of the dangers of smoking and therefore knowledge alone cannot explain individuals' behaviour. There appears to be a very complex interplay between several different factors. Graham (1993) identified that individuals continue to pursue unhealthy behaviours because of the potential benefits they provide. In her analysis of cigarette smoking among economically disadvantaged young mothers, she found individuals appeared to apply a process through which they weighed up the psychological benefits of smoking, such as stress release which served as an aid to calmer childcare, against the probability of physiological health damage and, in a reasoned and rational fashion, decided to continue to smoke.

> **ACTIVITY 3.4**
>
> Think about Graham's findings above and imagine working with a young mother who smokes around her children.
> - List some of the difficulties in suggesting she stop smoking.
> - List some principles from the Nursing and Midwifery Council's *Code* (NMC, 2018) that might aid your approach.

### 3.4.2 The materialist model

This model suggests that poverty has a direct impact on health; a position that is supported in Marmot's (2020) most recent review. Despite improvements in the overall standard of living across the UK, there are significant differences in the living conditions and personal circumstances of different social groups that may contribute to differences in their health experiences. Differences in work, housing, access to amenities and physical and social threats can directly impact on health (Sundmacher, Scheller-Kreinsen and Busse, 2011). The materialist model was favoured by the Black Report (Townsend, Davidson and Whitehead, 1988). However, there are factors that can mediate against the direct effects of financial deprivation, such as psychosocial factors including family and social support (Matthews, Gallo and Taylor, 2010).

### 3.4.3 Psychosocial model and the Spirit Level

The "Spirit Level" posed by Wilkinson and Pickett (2010) suggests that the greater the income inequality in a country, the greater the problems that society faces. They argue that inequality in society causes shorter, unhealthier, unhappier lives. For example, in societies where there is greater inequality, there are greater social problems and poorer health (Keeley, 2015) and the greater the inequality, the poorer the health (Marmot, 2015). Marmot (2015) cites the USA as an example of a wealthy country with excellent healthcare, but with extreme poverty and high mortality rates. The Spirit Level draws reference to the psychosocial model of health inequalities. This suggests that stressful situations such as poor living and working conditions can cause high blood pressure, development of diabetes and ischaemic heart disease. Such conditions can also influence health-related behaviours, such as drinking alcohol excessively, smoking, eating a poor diet and having limited physical activity (PHE, 2017b). Nurses, therefore, need to be aware of the complex relationship between social, economic and environmental factors and how they impact on each other in order to provide effective health promotion interventions.

### 3.4.4 Life-course model

According to Marmot (Marmot, 2010, 2020) disadvantage starts before birth. It influences a child's life chances and the impact accumulates throughout life. The life-course model recognises the behavioural and material influences on health along with the impact of mental wellbeing, stress and the control people can exercise over their health. Various aspects of the model are explored below and expanded upon in *Chapter 5*.

**Early years**

Social inequalities that impact on maternal health, such as diet, alcohol and stress, have a significant impact on foetal development. The early years, which are important for future physical and emotional development, are influenced by the distribution of resources, supportive family environments and parenting skills (National Academies of Sciences, Engineering and Medicine, 2016). The Welsh Adverse Childhood Experiences (ACE) Study (Public Health Wales, 2015) identified ACEs as stressful experiences occurring during childhood that directly harm a child (e.g. sexual or physical abuse) or affect the environment in which they live (e.g. growing up in a house with domestic violence). The study highlights that such experiences increase the risk of individuals developing health-harming behaviours in adult life.

> **ACTIVITY 3.5**
>
> List some approaches that may protect a child against future risk. Consider the role of the Family Nurse Partnership: https://fnp.nhs.uk.

**Education**

The educational achievement of a child is largely determined by their parents' social position, since this tends to influence parenting skills and primary socialisation. This, in turn, has an impact on the child's cognitive and emotional development. The parents' social position further impacts on characteristics such as perseverance, motivation, risk aversion and self-esteem, which all impact on a child's educational attainment (Marmot, 2020). The Joseph Rowntree Foundation (2014) found that the gap in reading ability between children from low-income and high-income households at the age of five years was approximately one year. In addition, parental socioeconomic background had a greater influence on educational attainment than the school attended, with children from deprived households leaving school earlier and less likely to enter higher education. The health visitor, children's nurse or the Family Nurse Partnership can have an important role in supporting families who experience deprivation, to promote a healthy start in life and provide a holistic upbringing.

**Education, employment and health**

The links between education and health have been identified by Ross and Wu (1995) and Miech *et al.* (2011). Educational attainment is one of the main determinants of income and employment. Well-educated people are more likely to be employed in full-time work and to have fulfilling, rewarding jobs with a higher income which, in turn, significantly improves health outcomes (Ross and Wu, 1995).

Better-educated people enjoy higher levels of social support and sense of control over health and life which, in turn, result in better physical and psychological health (Ross and Wu, 1995). Furthermore, the well-educated are more likely to exercise and less likely to smoke (Ross and Wu, 1995). Marmot (2010) highlights that people who are less well-educated are more likely to be in low-paid, poor-quality jobs with little opportunity for advancement. Such jobs frequently include activities that pose a risk to health, for example repetitive heavy lifting, as explored below. Marmot's (2020) more recent review reiterates these findings.

Emotional stability and the ability to establish social networks tend to be characteristics of the most well-educated and these have been found to be protective factors for health (Roberts *et al.*, 2007; Heckman and Kautz, 2012; Ver Ploeg, 2009). In contrast, men and women with less education tend to have smaller social networks (Antonucci, Ajrouch and Janevic, 2003; Marmot, 2010). Education builds skills and fosters traits such as conscientiousness, perseverance, self-control, problem solving, flexibility and the capacity for negotiation, all of which positively contribute towards health (OECD, 2015a). Limited access to education may mean that individuals do not have the opportunity to develop such traits, which renders them more vulnerable in relation to health. Nurses may sometimes come across children who are full-time carers and who are, therefore, missing out on their education. Nurses have a professional responsibility to protect those in their care (NMC, 2018) and should refer vulnerable children to social services.

The link between employment and health is also very close. Employment directly impacts on income, social networks, self-esteem and stress. Furthermore, the nature of work is closely associated with health. For example, adverse working conditions which are more prevalent in manual work can directly impact upon health by exposing individuals to physical hazards, long working shifts and musculoskeletal damage. Related complications such as low autonomy in work and workplace conflict can combine to create a toxic effect (Marmot *et al.*, 1997). Such factors are more prevalent in the most deprived workers where job security can be a concern and risk of unemployment is greater (PHE, 2015). Occupational health nurses have a role in protecting workers and advising on adjustments and health and safety in the workplace. However, it may be that some workers in the poorest paid or higher risk jobs do not have access to health services at work and illegal workers may be at particular risk.

### Income

The relationship between income and health is well known, with people with low incomes refraining from purchasing goods and services that maintain good health and being unable to afford to participate in many health-related activities (Marmot, 2010, 2020). Disadvantaged individuals often live in poor neighbourhoods with higher rates of unemployment, ill health and disability. These geographical areas are also likely to be the areas of deprivation identified earlier in the chapter. These communities are often marginalised and have more risk factors for poor health, such as limited access to supermarkets and an oversupply of fast food outlets that promote unhealthy diets (Burgoine *et al.*, 2014). Those with the lowest income are more likely to live in damp, temporary, overcrowded and insecure accommodation (Hitchman *et al.*, 2002).

> **ACTIVITY 3.6**
>
> Nurses have a special role in supporting people in poverty. Identify four available services to which nurses can signpost their patients.

## 3.5 Dis-/empowerment

Research by Marmot (2015) and Wilkinson and Pickett (2010) suggests that inequality affects not only those at the bottom of the social hierarchy (i.e. the most deprived), but everyone. A gradient exists where different levels of advantages and disadvantages are distributed across society, dependent on one's position. This means that those in the middle will have better health than those in the most deprived areas and worse health than those in the least deprived areas.

Recently, Marmot (2015, 2020) highlighted the damaging effect of disempowerment. The more disadvantaged a person or a whole community is, the more disempowered they are likely to feel. This creates barriers and denies access to resources that can make positive changes to people's lives and health. Where people lack finance, opportunity and structure to their lives, they become disempowered and make potentially unhealthy choices. Marmot (2015) describes three types of dis-/empowerment: material, psychosocial and political. He highlights *material disempowerment* as existing where there are insufficient financial resources to provide adequate food or shelter. *Psychosocial disempowerment* occurs where people do not have control over their lives to make decisions that would be beneficial to their overall health and wellbeing. *Political disempowerment* exists where there is an absence of a political voice or political party that creates policies that allocate necessary resources to improve the wellbeing of society. Marmot (2015) refers to Glasgow, where there is a 28-year difference in life expectancy between the wealthiest area of Lenzie and the most disadvantaged area of Carlton, which are only a few miles apart. Marmot suggests that this disempowerment is woven into the structure of society. An important role of the nurse is to empower people. This is particularly challenging when the people in the most deprived areas may be the most disempowered. But nurses can support people to take control over some parts of their lives and enable them to make the best decisions possible.

To improve the chances of a healthy life for individuals, in *Fair Society, Healthy Lives* Marmot (2010) outlines six policy objectives, with highest priority being given to the first:

1. giving every child the best start in life
2. enabling all children, young people and adults to maximise their capabilities and have control over their lives
3. creating fair employment and good work for all
4. ensuring a healthy standard of living for all
5. creating and developing sustainable places and communities
6. strengthening the role and impact of ill health prevention.

These policy objectives are reiterated in Marmot's 2020 review. They are particularly relevant for midwives, health visitors and nurses, who are at the front line of healthcare and see health inequalities first-hand. They are in a prime position to identify children who may be at risk and offer support to parents in making the best choices possible. Nurses can also make an impact by implementing MECC (PHE, 2018), as discussed in *Chapter 2*.

### CASE STUDY 3.1  DAWN'S STORY

Dawn lives on the tenth floor of a tower block in a disadvantaged area where there is gang culture, drug dealing and violent knife crime. Dawn's start in life was shaped by several adverse childhood events. She came from a single parent family where her mother had several male partners who treated both her and her mother badly. By the time Dawn started school she had behavioural problems. She left school with no qualifications, having become involved in gangs and violence.

Dawn is now aged 20 and is the single mother of two young children. With no role model she has difficulty making good choices for the children. Any money she makes goes on drink and cigarettes. She finds caring for her children challenging and uses the television and unhealthy snacks to control behaviour.

The lift in the tower block isn't working and Dawn doesn't have a car. So, when she needs to go shopping, she asks one of the neighbours to care for her children while she goes to the local supermarket to pick up convenience foods. However, the neighbour will often leave the children to go back to their own flat.

Dawn wants to work but can't afford to put her children in childcare. When she leaves them for short periods, she is worried that they may come to some harm. She lives from day to day, worrying about feeding her family and paying her bills. She is constantly hoping that she doesn't have to replace any of her white goods as she has no money and would need to borrow from a money lender. She and the children sleep and live in one room as it is too expensive to heat the whole flat.

Dawn's aspirations for her children are that they do not take drugs or end up in gangs. She knows that a mile down the road parents worry about which university their children can go to. Dawn has no such aspirations.

## ACTIVITY 3.7

Explore your own thoughts and ideas about Dawn and her situation. Do you have empathy for Dawn or do you feel frustrated that she spends her money on cigarettes and alcohol?

How might your own beliefs influence your approach to supporting Dawn?

## ACTIVITY 3.8

*Section 3.4* identifies some of the explanations for inequalities in health. Look back at the life-course theory in *Section 3.4.4* and identify how the following have impacted on Dawn's current situation:
- Early years
- Education
- Employment
- Income

How may the nurse be able to support Dawn in enhancing her health and the health of her children?

Most differences in health status can be explained by deprivation, but this is not the only cause. Inequalities in health are a complex interplay of factors; for example, there are differences in health status between men and women and between different ethnic groups. These are explored in the next sections of this chapter.

## 3.6 Gender differences in health

Gender refers to

> … *the array of socially constructed roles and relationships, personality traits, attitudes, behaviours, values, relative power and influence that society ascribes to the two sexes on a differential basis. Gender is relational – gender roles and characteristics do not exist in isolation, but are defined in relation to one another and through the relationships between women and men, girls and boys.*
>
> (Health Canada, 2000, p. 14)

In other words, sex refers to biological differences, whereas gender refers to social differences.

Women live longer than men (Annandale, 2014) but experience more years in poor health (White, 2017). In addition to overall mortality and morbidity, certain health and wellbeing issues are more commonly associated with a particular gender. For example, dementia, depression and arthritis are more common in women (Weber *et al.*, 2019) and women are more likely to be subject to physical and emotional violence (Barry and Yuill, 2016). Men, on the other hand, are more prone to lung cancer, cardiovascular disease and suicide (WHO, 2019).

Biological differences alone cannot adequately explain gender-based health differences or health behaviour. The following section will explore some of the social factors that contribute to gender differences in health and behaviour.

> **ACTIVITY 3.9**
>
> Have you considered that you or your friends may participate in social roles and activities that are characterised by gender? When you read the section below, consider whether any of this rings true for you.

### 3.6.1 Early socialisation

Children learn and adopt behaviours through observing their parents or carers and through play. Parents can instil and reinforce gender-based behaviours by promoting certain forms of play or clothing, praising or punishing types of behaviour and modelling behaviours such as housework or DIY. In turn, these actions can influence children's choices in later life, including gender-based beliefs about future work success (Bornstein, Putnick and Lansford, 2011; Bussey and Bandura, 1999).

> **ACTIVITY 3.10**
>
> Consider how early socialisation may impact on education and employment.
>
> Can you see how this may have an impact on health?

### 3.6.2 Education

The OECD (2015b) reports differences in achievement and attitudes towards education between boys and girls. Girls do better in school than boys, with 15-year-old boys less likely to achieve a baseline level of proficiency in reading, mathematics and science. Girls demonstrate better behaviour in class and spend more time on homework and reading outside of school. However, in high-achieving students we see a difference within the science subjects, with girls at 15 years doing less well in mathematics, science and problem solving compared to their male peers. Even when boys and girls are equally proficient in mathematics and science, their attitudes towards learning and aspirations for their future are markedly different. Girls report stronger feelings of anxiety towards mathematics than boys. In turn, greater mathematics anxiety is associated with a decline in performance, leading to different subject choices, which impacts upon choice of career. Wang (2012) found that girls perceived teachers as being more interested in teaching boys and this subsequently demotivated them. For example, women are far more likely than men to study subjects relating to education, teaching, health and the social sector (and are subsequently over-represented in these professions). Men, on the other hand, are more likely to choose science or engineering which, in turn, lead to higher salaries in the labour market.

## 3.6.3 Employment

In *Section 3.4.4* we saw that income can have a direct effect on health. Women earn less than men, with men at the age of 49 years earning an average of 45% more than women (ONS, 2014). There are several reasons for this: men's choice of job can earn them a better income and women may choose to work part-time to care for children. However, Barry and Yuill (2016) argue that women in the UK can find themselves trapped between 'sticky floors' and 'glass ceilings', which means because of discrimination women may be more likely to stay at the lower grades and not achieve the same promotion opportunities as men.

Gendered roles not only have an impact on earning potential, they can also impact upon the nature of employment. Women are more likely to take parental leave, work part-time or flexibly and to work in the informal sector, resulting in a lower income (Kings College London, 2019). Women are the main providers of informal care for children, disabled and older people. The effects of this role can include reduced sleep, less leisure time and increased risk of poverty for women who are full-time carers. All these factors can have serious negative consequences for both physical and mental health. Indeed, it has been suggested that the potential impact of the caring role on mental wellbeing may explain the higher rates of depression in women of childbearing age (Biaggi *et al.*, 2016). Men, on the other hand, are more likely to find themselves in employment that is dangerous, for example working with dangerous machinery, environmental hazards, exposure to toxic chemicals and in extreme weather (Scambler, 2012).

## 3.6.4 Health behaviours

Health behaviours also vary between males and females. Men are more likely to engage in risk-taking behaviour than women; for example, they are more likely to take part in contact sports, drink excessive alcohol and drive recklessly. As a result, males have higher rates of accidental and non-accidental injuries (Fisk, 2018).

Wang, Eccles and Kenny (2013) and White (2017) found differences in attendance at GP clinics and hospitals across the genders, with men attending less than women. Some of the differences in attendance have been attributed to women requiring more access to healthcare; for example, for contraception, screening programmes for cervical cancer and maternity services. However, it may also be because men are less likely to communicate their health needs and are reluctant to ask for help (O'Brien, Hart and Hunt, 2007; Wang, Eccles and Kenny, 2013).

> **ACTIVITY 3.11**
>
> Consider how your role in promoting health may differ between men and women.
>
> How may you need to change your approach for different genders?
>
> Might there be different motivating and enabling factors for men and women?

Chapter 3: Inequalities in health

## 3.7 Gender fluidity

Gender and gender identification extend beyond traditional male and female identities. Generally, LGBTQ (lesbian, gay, bisexual, transgender and queer/questioning) people tend to identify as male or female. More recently, there has been increasing recognition and visibility of people who do not identify exclusively as either male or female. Non-binary gender identity is an identity that does not categorise as either man or woman. Other terms that non-binary individuals will use to identify themselves as are *genderqueer*, *agender* and *bigender*.

LGBTQ and non-binary individuals experience a number of different health issues. Scandura *et al.* (2019) identify that people who don't conform to traditional gender identities often become targets of discrimination, leading to negative mental health issues. This may be because there is a lack of knowledge and information about this population. However, non-binary individuals may also have more difficulty in the process of recognition of identity (coming out) due to a lack of visibility of this population (Tebbe and Moradi, 2016), leading to greater risk of mental health issues such as anxiety and depression (James *et al.*, 2016). In addition, Booker, Rieger and Unger (2017) found that gay, lesbian and bisexual individuals had worse physical health and were more likely to smoke, drink alcohol and take drugs.

Inequalities are also evident in accessing healthcare. The Government Equalities Office's (2018) research on the experiences of the LGBTQ community identified that at least 16% of their respondents who accessed public health services had a negative experience because of their sexual orientation, and at least 38% had a negative experience because of their gender identity. Of those trying to access mental health services, 51% said they had to wait too long, 27% were worried, anxious or embarrassed about going and 16% said their GP was not supportive. Of the transgender respondents who tried to access gender identity clinics, 80% said it was not easy, with long waiting times the most common barrier. The LGBT foundation (Williams *et al.*, 2010) also identified that this community were less likely to take advantage of screening programmes; this may be explained by Lykens, LeBlanc and Bockting (2018) and Baldwin *et al.* (2018) in identifying that health professionals can be unfamiliar with the identity and needs of non-binary individuals. Non-binary individuals frequently feel misunderstood by providers, who often approach them as male or female (Lykens, LeBlanc and Bockting, 2018) and experience negative interactions because of unfamiliarity with identity and health issues (Baldwin *et al.*, 2018).

As nurses we have a specific role in supporting people with non-traditional genders in our care. The Equality Act (HM Government, 2010) ensures that vulnerable and minority groups are protected legally. As a profession we should take steps to meet the needs of people who have characteristics that are different from the majority. There are a number of measures that we as nurses can take that can make the healthcare experience more positive. Being non-judgemental, respectful and supportive is a basic requirement identified by the NMC (2018) for all patients and

The National Centre for Transgender Equality (2018) offers specific guidelines for non-binary individuals.

> **ACTIVITY 3.12**
>
> Think about a person who has female sex organs but identifies as male or non-binary. How might they feel attending a women's health clinic for a Pap smear or attending a breast clinic?
>
> Equally, how might someone with male sex organs who now identifies as a woman feel if they were an inpatient on a male urology ward?

Some of the actions you may have considered in *Activity 3.12* may have required you to think quite differently about how we organise health services. We can do several things to make such situations easier, for example by providing gender-neutral waiting rooms, not referring to clinics as male or female clinics and offering non-binary/transgender people specific times for appointments or single rooms on wards.

## 3.8 Ethnicity and health

Bartley (2017) suggests that race relates to biological or genetic differences between people, whereas ethnicity is a complex mix of biology, culture, lifestyle, religion and language. There is a growing body of evidence documenting ethnic inequalities in health outcomes in the UK. However, measuring health outcomes amongst different ethnicities is problematic. There can be as many variations within ethnic groups as there are between ethnic groups. For example, the term 'south Asian' will include populations from Bangladesh, India, Pakistan and Sri Lanka, with each of these countries having different cultural behaviours. Furthermore, ethnicity is not recorded on UK death certificates and mortality data uses country of birth as a proxy, thus failing to identify ethnic minorities born in the UK.

> **ACTIVITY 3.13**
>
> Define your race and ethnicity. Consider some of your health choices – are they determined by your ethnicity?

Migrants to Britain have different experiences of health and ill health. Men and women born in the Caribbean have high rates of mortality from stroke and individuals born in west/southern Africa have high overall mortality rates. Individuals born in south Asia have high mortality rates from coronary heart disease and stroke (PHE, 2017c). Between 1991 and 2011 Pakistani and Bangladeshi women had mortality rates 10% higher than white women (Becares, 2013). In 2011, men from white Gypsy or Irish Traveller minority groups, along with mixed white-black Caribbean men, white Irish men and black Caribbean men, all had higher rates of long-term illness than white men (Becares, 2013). Long-term illness in men aged over 65 years was reported by 69% of white Gypsy or Irish Traveller men, 69% of Pakistani men and 64% of Bangladeshi men, compared with 50% of white men. The Chinese group within the study reported persistently better health in both men and women compared to the white majority (Becares, 2013).

These health disparities stem from economic determinants, education, geography and neighbourhood environment (e.g. access to healthy food outlets and recreational facilities, air and noise pollution) and the chronic stress that arises from poverty and discrimination (Bahls, 2011). The fourth national survey on ethnic minorities in Britain was a major study that has yet to be replicated (Nazroo, 1997, 2001). It showed that ethnic minorities had lower incomes, poorer quality housing and were unemployed longer than their white counterparts (Rechel *et al.*, 2013). The relative deprivation faced by people of different ethnic backgrounds is likely to involve more than material disadvantage. For example, individuals face marginalisation, alienation and racial harassment.

In order to understand the differences in health status amongst different ethnic groups, we need to understand what individuals experience in the process of migration, education and employment. This is discussed below.

### 3.8.1 Migration

We live in an increasingly globalised world, where individuals and families are moving from one country to another. The UN (2015) has identified a significant increase in international migration over recent years, reaching 244 million in 2015. There are a variety of different reasons for migration, and migration is often split into two categories: *voluntary migration*, such as employment opportunities and quality of life factors, and *forced migration*, such as war, poverty, political and economic instability or trafficking. It is important to recognise that migrant groups are very diverse and the impact of migration on health will be different for different groups of migrants (Juhász, Makara and Taller, 2010).

While migration can have a positive effect on health, it is also known to influence health negatively in several ways. For example, Rechel *et al.* (2013) identify that migrant groups are more susceptible to certain communicable diseases (e.g. tuberculosis (TB)), occupational health hazards, injuries, obesity-related conditions, poor maternal and child health and mental health conditions. Rechel *et al.* (2013) suggest that the greatest impact on health for migrants is deprivation. Migrants are more at risk of poor living conditions, overcrowding and homelessness (Migration Observatory, 2019); they are susceptible to poor working conditions and are overrepresented in low qualified and temporary high-risk jobs (OECD, 2017). Lifestyle factors are also a concern, as migrants adopt the high calorie western diet and sedentary lifestyle, leading to weight-related conditions. Furthermore, migrants find difficulty accessing and navigating the healthcare system. In part, this is attributable to language difficulties (Pace, 2011; Norredam, Nielsen and Krasnik, 2010) which can increase the risk of persistent poverty (Fisher and Nandi, 2015) and poor health. Undocumented migrants are at greatest risk of deprivation as they are the most marginalised in society (Rechel *et al.*, 2013). It is therefore important that nurses minimise barriers to access; this might involve language support, outreach work and trying to provide health promotion through alternative channels such as schools or communities.

> **ACTIVITY 3.14**
>
> Consider how you might need to change your approach if you are promoting the health of an individual who may be a new migrant to the UK. Think about how their priorities may be different from yours.
>
> Imagine you are a health visitor caring for a family from Pakistan; they consist of a mum at 22 years old, dad at 24 and two young children who are 10 months and 3 years. They share a house with three other families and there is no income as the dad doesn't work.
>
> What do you think the family's priorities may be?
>
> What might the social and health risks be for this family?
>
> What would be your priorities?

It is important to note, however, that inequalities are not only evident amongst migrants. British-born people from black, Asian, minority ethnic (BAME) groups in the UK face greater inequalities in income and health than the white majority. They live in the most deprived areas (as measured by the indices of deprivation (see *Section 3.2*), which are populated with approximately four times more BAME people than more affluent areas (Brown, Bramley and Watkins, 2010). Public Health England (2019) recognises the specific need of BAME people living in deprivation and suggests that geographical areas should be targeted with an attempt to address the policy directives outlined by Marmot in *Section 3.5*. They also suggest strengthening community action, which is discussed in *Chapter 8*. Nurses working in these geographical areas benefit from having cultural awareness.

## 3.8.2 Education

The experience of BAME groups in education is a complex one. For some, initial language barriers mean that children start school at a disadvantage, but they quickly catch up with their white peers. BAME groups generally do well in secondary education. They tend to stay on longer in full-time education, show a greater commitment to study and achieve higher grades (Li, Devine and Heath, 2008). Indian and Chinese children continue to outperform all ethnic groups at all key stages (Eden, 2017). This, Li, Devine and Heath (2008) explain, is because they recognise that education is essential for economic success. However, while higher numbers of BAME groups are now entering higher education (HEFCE, 2018), Universities UK and the National Union of Students (2019) identified that ethnic groups do not do so well in higher education, with lower proportions of BAME students in the most prestigious universities than their white counterparts. Analysis by the Office for Students (2019) shows that with the exception of students of Chinese heritage, more BAME students discontinue their studies compared with their white peers, and more black students discontinue their studies than any other ethnic group. Their analysis also shows that fewer BAME students achieve a first-class degree or a 2:1 than their white peers.

Education is often seen as the route out of poverty, but being successful in education does not always result in success in employment for BAME groups: 40% of African and 39% of Bangladeshi graduates are overqualified for the jobs they work in and they are less likely to get a good return for university education, compared to their white colleagues (Brynin and Longhi, 2015).

### 3.8.3 Employment

The picture for employment shows similar patterns of inequality to those described above. In 2018 the employment rate in the UK was higher for the white majority (77%) compared with all other ethnic groups combined (65%) (ONS, 2018). Ethnic groups more likely to experience unemployment were white Gypsy/Irish Traveller groups and Pakistani and Bangladeshi groups. This appears to be linked to women from these groups undertaking unpaid caring responsibilities in the home (Nazroo and Kapadia, 2013; ONS, 2018).

Amongst those who are employed, certain BAME groups are likely to earn significantly less than their white counterparts. There is a greater likelihood of working in low-paid jobs that have very little prospect of progression and Bangladeshi workers are the most likely to earn below the living wage and to be the lowest paid, regardless of the area they work in. The Joseph Rowntree Foundation (2017) argues that much of this is explained by racism and discrimination. All this contributes to rates of poverty and as this chapter has highlighted, poverty has a negative impact on health.

Because those in worst health are likely to come from the most deprived backgrounds that include people from BAME backgrounds, it is crucial that we as nurses make an effort to understand the social context in which people live and develop a cultural awareness of the needs of the population we care for.

## 3.9 Social change

Returning to *Chapter 2*, Scriven (2017) highlights medical, empowerment, educational, behavioural and social change processes as central to supporting behavioural change. In the context of inequalities in health, a consideration of social change is essential. Marmot (2015, p. 1) asks, *"why treat people and send them back to the conditions that made them sick?"*. Baum and Fisher (2014) suggest that health promotion strategies alone are ineffective and there needs to be policy to reduce inequality to improve education, housing, employment, income and wealth. They suggest redistributing resources to narrow the inequality gap. Nurses have a voice in lobbying for social change. We can also make a difference by signposting individuals and families to other members of the multidisciplinary team who are well-placed in supporting people to access financial support, education, housing and employment.

## KEY LEARNING POINTS

Four key points to take away from *Chapter 3*:
- Inequalities in health are evident throughout society, with those at the lower end of the social hierarchy facing the worst health, regardless of their gender or ethnicity.
- Inequalities in health are underpinned by a complex interplay between contributing factors.
- Any activity aimed at improving health status must account for the challenges faced by people with the worst health.
- Social change is an essential aspect of health promotion.

# REFERENCES

Acheson, D. (1988) *Independent Inquiry into Inequalities in Health Report*. Available at: https://assets.publishing.service.gov.uk/government/uploads/system/uploads/attachment_data/file/265503/ih.pdf (accessed 6 May 2020)

Annandale, E. (2014) *The Sociology of Health and Medicine: a critical introduction*, 2nd edition. Polity Press.

Antonucci, T., Ajrouch, K. and Janevic, M. (2003) The effects of social relations with children on the education–health link in men and women aged 40 and over. *Social Science and Medicine*, **56(5):** 949–60.

Bahls, C. (2011) Achieving Equity in Health. *Health Policy Brief*. Available at: www.healthaffairs.org/healthpolicybriefs/brief.php?brief_id=53 (accessed 11 May 2020)

Baldwin, A., Dodge, B., Schick, V. *et al*. (2018) Transgender and genderqueer individuals' experiences with health care providers: what's working, what's not, and where do we go from here? *Journal of Health Care for the Poor and Underserved*, **29(4):** 1300–18.

Barry, A-M. and Yuill, C. (2016) *Understanding the Sociology of Health*, 4th edition. SAGE.

Bartley, M. (2017) *Health Inequality: an introduction to concepts, theories and methods*, 2nd edition. Polity Press.

Baum, F. and Fisher, M. (2014) Why behavioural health promotion endures despite its failure to reduce health inequities. *Sociology of Health and Illness*, **36(2):** 213–25.

Becares, L. (2013) *Which ethnic groups have the poorest health?* Available at: http://hummedia.manchester.ac.uk/institutes/code/briefingsupdated/which-ethnic-groups-have-the-poorest-health.pdf (accessed 11 May 2020)

Biaggi, A., Conroy, S., Pawlby, S. and Pariante, C. (2016) Identifying the women at risk of antenatal anxiety and depression: a systematic review. *Journal of Affective Disorders*, **191:** 62–77. DOI: 10.1016/j.jad.2015.11.014.

Booker, C., Rieger, G. and Unger, J. (2017) Sexual orientation health inequality: evidence from *Understanding Society*, the UK Longitudinal Household Study. *Preventive Medicine*, **101:** 126–32. Available at https://doi.org/10.1016/j.ypmed.2017.06.010 (accessed 7 July 2020)

Bornstein, M., Putnick, D. and Lansford, J. (2011) Parenting attributions and attitudes in cross-cultural perspective. *Parenting Science and Practice*, **11(2–3):** 214–37.

Brown, C., Bramley, G. and Watkins, D. (2010) *Urban Green Nation: building the evidence base*. Commission for Architecture and the Built Environment (CABE).

Brynin, M. and Longhi, S. (2015) *The Effect of Occupation on Poverty Among Ethnic Minority Groups*. Joseph Rowntree Foundation.

Burgoine, T., Forouhi, N., Griffin, S., Wareham, N. and Monsivais, P. (2014) Associations between exposure to takeaway food outlets, takeaway food consumption, and body weight in Cambridgeshire, UK: population based, cross sectional study. *BMJ*, **348:** g1464. DOI: https://doi.org/10.1136/bmj.g1464

Bussey, K. and Bandura, A. (1999) Social cognitive theory of gender development and differentiation. *Psychological Review*, **106(4):** 676–713.

Eden, C. (2017) *Gender, Education and Work: inequalities and intersectionality*. Routledge.

Fisher, P. and Nandi, A. (2015) *Poverty Across Ethnic Groups Through Recession and Austerity*. Joseph Rowntree Foundation.

Fisk, S. (2018) Who's on top? Gender differences in risk-taking produce unequal outcomes for high-ability women and men. *Social Psychology Quarterly*, **81(3):** 185–206.

Government Equalities Office (2018) *LGBT Action Plan*. Available at: https://assets.publishing.service.gov.uk/government/uploads/system/uploads/attachment_data/file/721367/GEO-LGBT-Action-Plan.pdf (accessed 11 May 2020)

Graham, H. (1993) *Hardship and Health in Women's Lives*. Routledge.

Health Canada (2000) *Health Canada's Gender-based Analysis Policy*. Health Canada.

Heckman, J. and Kautz, T. (2012) Hard evidence on soft skills. *Labour Economics*, **19(4):** 451–64.

HEFCE (2018) *Differences in Student Outcomes: the effect of student characteristics*. Available at: https://webarchive.nationalarchives.gov.uk/20180405115303/http://www.hefce.ac.uk/pubs/year/2018/201805/ (accessed 11 May 2020)

Hernandez, J. and Kim, P. (2020) *Epidemiology Morbidity and Mortality*. In: StatPearls (internet). Available at: www.ncbi.nlm.nih.gov/books/NBK547668/ (accessed 11 May 2020)

Hitchman, C., Christie, I., Harrison, M. and Lang, T. (2002) *Inconvenience Food: the struggle to eat well on a low income*. Available at: www.demos.co.uk/files/inconveniencefood.pdf (accessed 11 May 2020)

HM Government (2010) Equality Act 2010. Available at: www.legislation.gov.uk/ukpga/2010/15 (accessed 11 May 2020)

Institute of Health Equity (2018) *Launching 2020: the Marmot Review 10 years on*. Available at: www.health.org.uk/news-and-comment/news/health-equity-in-england-the-marmot-review-10-years-on (accessed 11 May 2020)

James, S., Herman, J., Rankin, S. et al. (2016) *The Report of the 2015 U.S. Transgender Survey*. National Center for Transgender Equality.

Joseph Rowntree Foundation (2014) *Closing the Attainment Gap in Scottish Education*. Available at: https://www.jrf.org.uk/report/closing-attainment-gap-scottish-education (accessed 11 May 2020)

Joseph Rowntree Foundation (2017) *Poverty and Ethnicity in the Labour Market*. Available at: www.jrf.org.uk/report/poverty-ethnicity-labour-market (accessed 11 May 2020)

Juhász, J., Makara, P. and Taller, A. (2010) *Possibilities and Limitations of Comparative Research on International Migration and Health*. PROMINSTAT / European Commission.

Keeley, B. (2015) *Income Inequality: the gap between rich and poor*. OECD Publishing. Available at: https://doi.org/10.1787/9789264246010-6-en (accessed 11 May 2020)

King's Fund (2020) *What are Health Inequalities?* Available at: www.kingsfund.org.uk/publications/what-are-health-inequalities (accessed 11 May 2020)

Kings College London (2019) *Women's Progression in the Workplace*. Available at: www.kcl.ac.uk/giwl/assets/womens-progression-in-the-workplace.pdf (accessed 11 May 2020)

Li, Y., Devine, F. and Heath, A. (2008) *Equality Group Inequalities in Education, Employment and Earnings: a research review and analysis of trends over time*. EHRC.

Lykens J., LeBlanc A. and Bockting, W. (2018) Healthcare experiences among young adults who identify as genderqueer or nonbinary. *LGBT Health*, **5(3):** 191–6.

Marmot, M. (2010) *Fair Society, Healthy Lives*. Available at: www.parliament.uk/documents/fair-society-healthy-lives-full-report.pdf (accessed 6 May 2020)

Marmot, M. (2015) *The Health Gap: the challenge of an unequal world*. Bloomsbury.

Marmot, M. (2020) *Health Equity in England: the Marmot review 10 years on*. Institute of Health Equity. Available at: www.health.org.uk/sites/default/files/upload/publications/2020/Health%20Equity%20in%20England_The%20Marmot%20Review%2010%20Years%20On_full%20report.pdf (accessed 6 May 2020)

Marmot, M., Smith, G., Stansfeld, S. et al. (1991) Health inequalities among British civil servants: the Whitehall II study. *Lancet*, **337(8754):** 1387–93.

Marmot, M., Bosma, H., Hemingway, H., Brunner, E. and Stansfeld, S. (1997) Contribution of job control and other risk factors to social variations in coronary heart disease incidence. *Lancet*, **350(9073):** 235–9.

Matthews, K., Gallo, L. and Taylor, S. (2010) Are psychosocial factors mediators of socioeconomic status and health connections? A progress report and blueprint for the future. *Annals of the New York Academy of Sciences*, **1186:** 146–73.

Miech, R., Pampel, F., Kim, J. and Rogers, R. (2011) The enduring association between education and mortality: the role of widening and narrowing disparities. *American Sociological Review*, **76(6):** 913–34.

Migration Observatory (2019) Available at: https://migrationobservatory.ox.ac.uk/resources/briefings/migrants-and-housing-in-the-uk-experiences-and-impacts/ (accessed 11 May 2020)

National Academies of Sciences, Engineering, and Medicine (2016) *Parenting Matters: supporting parents of children ages 0–8*. The National Academies Press.

National Centre for Transgender Equality (2018) *Understanding Non-Binary People: How to Be Respectful and Supportive*. Available at: https://transequality.org/issues/resources/understanding-non-binary-people-how-to-be-respectful-and-supportive (accessed 30 January 2020)

Nazroo, J. (1997) *The Health of Britain's Ethnic Minorities*. Policy Studies Institute.

Nazroo, J. (2001) *Ethnicity, Class and Health* (PSI Research Report 880). Policy Studies Institute.

Nazroo, J. and Kapadia, D. (2013) *Ethnic inequalities in labour market participation? Dynamic of diversity: Evidence from the 2011 Census*. The University of Manchester.

Norredam, M., Nielsen, S. and Krasnik, A. (2010) Migrants' utilization of somatic healthcare services in Europe—a systematic review. *European Journal of Public Health*, **20(5):** 555–63.

Nursing and Midwifery Council (2018) *The Code: professional standards of practice and behaviour for nurses, midwives and nursing associates*. NMC.

O'Brien, R., Hart, G. and Hunt, K. (2007) "Standing out from the herd": men renegotiating masculinity in relation to their experience of illness. *International Journal of Men's Health*, **6(3):** 178–200.

OECD (2015a) *Skills for Social Progress: the power of social and emotional skills*. Available at: http://dx.doi.org/10.1787/9789264226159-en (accessed 11 May 2020)

OECD (2015b) *The ABC of Gender Equality in Education*. Available at: http://dx.doi.org/10.1787/9789264229945-en (accessed 11 May 2020)

OECD (2017) *Migrants' Well-being: moving to a better life?* Available at: www.oecd-ilibrary.org/sites/how_life-2017-7-en/index.html?itemId=/content/component/how_life-2017-7-en (accessed 11 May 2020)

Office for Students (2019) *Ethnicity*. Available at: www.officeforstudents.org.uk/advice-and-guidance/promoting-equal-opportunities/evaluation-and-effective-practice/ethnicity/ (accessed 11 May 2020)

ONS (2014) *UK Wages Over the Past Four Decades*. Available at: https://data.gov.uk/dataset/60552637-3991-4cde-bd0f-21937f7da8bd/uk-wages-over-the-past-four-decades (accessed 11 May 2020)

ONS (2018) *Ethnicity Pay Gaps in Great Britain: 2018*. Available at: www.ons.gov.uk/employmentandlabourmarket/peopleinwork/earningsandworkinghours/articles/ethnicitypaygapsingreatbritain/2018#main-points (accessed 11 May 2020)

ONS (2019) *Health State Life Expectancies by National Deprivation Deciles, England and Wales: 2015 to 2017*. Available at: www.ons.gov.uk/peoplepopulationandcommunity/healthandsocialcare/healthinequalities/bulletins/healthstatelifeexpectanciesbyindexofmultipledeprivationimd/2015to2017 (accessed 13 January 2020)

Pace, P. (2011) 'The right to health of migrants in Europe'. In Rechel, B., Mladovsky, P., Devillé, W. et al. (eds) *Migration and Health in the European Union*. Open University Press.

Public Health England (2015) *Local Action on Health Inequalities: promoting good quality jobs to reduce health inequalities*. Available at: https://assets.publishing.service.gov.uk/government/

# References

uploads/system/uploads/attachment_data/file/460700/2a_Promoting_good_quality_jobs-Full.pdf (accessed 11 May 2020)

Public Health England (2017a) *Chapter 5: Inequality in Health*. Available at: www.gov.uk/government/publications/health-profile-for-england/chapter-5-inequality-in-health (accessed 11 May 2020)

Public Health England (2017b) *Psychosocial Pathways and Health Outcomes: informing action on health inequalities*. Available at: www.instituteofhealthequity.org/resources-reports/psychosocial-pathways-and-health-outcomes-informing-action-on-health-inequalities/psychosocial-pathways-and-health-outcomes.pdf (accessed 11 May 2020)

Public Health England (2017c) *Public Health Outcomes Framework: Health Equity Report. Focus on ethnicity*. Available at: https://assets.publishing.service.gov.uk/government/uploads/system/uploads/attachment_data/file/733093/PHOF_Health_Equity_Report.pdf (accessed 11 May 2020)

Public Health England (2018) *Making Every Contact Count (MECC): implementation guide*. Available at: https://assets.publishing.service.gov.uk/government/uploads/system/uploads/attachment_data/file/769488/MECC_Implememenation_guide_v2.pdf (accessed 11 May 2020)

Public Health England (2019) *Health Inequalities: place-based approaches to reduce inequalities*. Available at: www.gov.uk/government/publications/health-inequalities-place-based-approaches-to-reduce-inequalities (accessed 11 May 2020)

Public Health Wales (2015) *Welsh Adverse Childhood Experiences (ACE) Study. Adverse Childhood Experiences and their impact on health-harming behaviours in the Welsh adult population*. Available at: http://researchonline.ljmu.ac.uk/id/eprint/2648/1/ACE%20Report%20FINAL%20%28E%29.pdf (accessed 11 May 2020)

Rechel, B., Mladovsky, P., Ingleby, D., Mackenbach, J. and McKee, M. (2013) Migration and health in an increasingly diverse Europe. *Lancet*, **381(9873):** 1235–45.

Roberts, B., Kuncel, N., Shine, R., Caspi, A. and Goldberg, L. (2007) The power of personality: the comparative validity of personality traits, socioeconomic status and cognitive ability for predicting important life outcomes. *Perspectives on Psychological Science*, **2(4):** 313–45.

Ross, C. and Wu, C-L. (1995) The links between education and health. *American Sociological Review*, **60(5):** 719–45.

Sanderson, M., Aldrich, M., Levine, R. *et al.* (2018) Neighbourhood deprivation and lung cancer risk: a nested case-control study in the USA. *BMJ Open*, **8(9):** e021059.

Scambler, G. (2012) Health inequalities. *Sociology of Health and Illness*, **34(1):** 130–46.

Scandura, C., Mezza, F., Maldonato, N. *et al.* (2019) Health of non-binary and genderqueer people: a systematic review. *Frontiers in Psychology*, DOI: 10.3389/fpsyg.2019.01453.

Scriven, A. (2017) *Ewles & Simnett's Promoting Health: a practical guide*, 7th edition. Elsevier.

Stait, E. and Calnan, M. (2016) Are differential consumption patterns in health-related behaviours an explanation for persistent and widening social inequalities in health in England? *International Journal for Equity in Health*, **15(171):** DOI:10.1186/s12939-016-0461-2.

Sundmacher, L., Scheller-Kreinsen, D. and Busse, R. (2011) The wider determinants of inequalities in health: a decomposition analysis. *International Journey for Equity in Health*, **10(30):** DOI:10.1186/1475-9276-10-30.

Tebbe, E. and Moradi, B. (2016) Suicide risk in trans populations: an application of minority stress theory. *Journal of Counselling Psychology*, **63(5):** 520–33.

Townsend, P., Davidson, N. and Whitehead, M. (1988) *Inequalities in Health: the Black Report and the health divide*. Pelican.

United Nations (2015) *International Migration Report 2015: highlights*. Available at: www.un.org/en/development/desa/population/migration/publications/migrationreport/docs/MigrationReport2015_Highlights.pdf (accessed 11 May 2020)

Universities UK and National Union of Students (2019) *Black, Asian and Minority Ethnic Student Attainment at UK Universities: #Closingthe gap*. Available at: www.universitiesuk.ac.uk/policy-and-analysis/reports/Documents/2019/bame-student-attainment-uk-universities-closing-the-gap.pdf (accessed 11 May 2020)

Ver Ploeg, M. (2009) *Access to affordable and nutritious food: measuring and understanding food deserts and their consequences*. Report to Congress. United States Department of Agriculture.

Wang, M-T. (2012) Educational and career interests in math: a longitudinal examination of the links between perceived classroom environment, motivational beliefs, and interests. *Developmental Psychology*, **48(6):** 1643–57.

Wang, M-T., Eccles, J. and Kenny, S. (2013) Not lack of ability but more choice: individual and gender differences in choice of careers in sciences, technology, engineering, and mathematics. *Psychological Science*, **24(5):** 770–5.

Weber, A., Mak, S., Berenbaum, F. *et al.* (2019) Association between osteoarthritis and increased risk of dementia. A systematic review and meta analysis. Medicine, **98(10):** 14355 DOI: 10.1097/MD.0000000000014355.

White, K. (2017) *An Introduction to the Sociology of Health and Illness*, 2nd edition. SAGE.

Wilkinson, R. and Pickett, K. (2010) *The Spirit Level: why equality is better for everyone*. Penguin.

Williams, H., Varney, J., Taylor, J. *et al.* (2010) *LGBT Public Health Outcomes Framework Companion Document*. Available at: www.london.gov.uk/sites/default/files/LGBT%20Public%20Health%20Outcomes%20Framework%20Companion%20Doc.pdf (accessed 11 May 2020)

WHO (2006) *Life Expectancy at Birth*. Available at: www.who.int/whosis/whostat2006DefinitionsAndMetadata.pdf (accessed 11 May 2020)

WHO (2019) *World Health Statistics Overview 2019. Monitoring health for the SDGs*. Available at: https://apps.who.int/iris/bitstream/handle/10665/311696/WHO-DAD-2019.1-eng.pdf (accessed 11 May 2020)

# Chapter 4
# Global health and wellbeing

Michelle Moseley

> **LEARNING OUTCOMES**
>
> When you have finished this chapter, you should be able to:
>
> 4.1 Discuss global public health and the UN sustainable development goals
>
> 4.2 Define epidemiology and consider how health is measured
>
> 4.3 Define genomics and explore its relevance in public health
>
> 4.4 Outline how the social determinants of health impact public health practice.

## 4.1 Introduction

This chapter will focus on the impact of global health directives that aim to improve the health and wellbeing of populations. In order to do this, there will be signposting to the sustainable development goals, an exploration of epidemiology and a discussion concerning the importance of genomics in public health. How we measure health will be addressed, particularly within the epidemiology section of the chapter. The wider and social determinants of health will also be discussed due to their relevance in the uptake of health promotion interventions.

## 4.2 Definitions and rationale

Global health and wellbeing refer to a worldwide partnership response to global health matters, with the aim of improving global population health and wellbeing physically, psychologically and environmentally. This is driven by the UN General Assembly and the WHO, who endorsed the seventeen sustainable development goals (UN General Assembly, 2015) outlined in *Figure 4.1*. Global health is relevant to all and is influenced by politics, finances, health equity and the environment (Sethia and Kumar, 2019). Global health is defined as *"a distinct entity... evolved from the study of public health, tropical medicine, and international health"* and is underpinned by the process of globalisation and its impact on the economic environment, health systems and the health of people, communities and countries (Eliasz, 2019, p. 2).

*Chapter 4: Global health and wellbeing*

Population health and wellbeing is at the heart of global public health and, therefore, relates to the improvement of health and wellbeing of individuals. Globalisation refers to how well connected nations are in the 21st century. This can have a positive influence on the delivery of health services, if accessible, due to greater mobility of staff and service users, worldwide availability of health service providers and access to advanced technology (Abdalla and Ognenis, 2019).

> **ACTIVITY 4.1**
>
> - Make a list of the major global health challenges today.
> - Compare your list to that on the WHO's website: www.who.int

The WHO and UN are key players in promoting the end to poverty, protecting the planet and improving the general health and wellbeing of individuals worldwide. In 2015 the UN General Assembly published the sustainable development goals and these were adopted by UN member states across the world. The aim is to achieve the goals within 15 years and by the year 2030, with climate change as a major target (UN General Assembly, 2015). In 2019, the Sustainable Development Goal (SDG) summit placed an emphasis on the next ten years in reaching the 2030 target (UN, 2019). The goals are all public health challenges and they underpin member states' public health priorities.

> **ACTIVITY 4.2**
>
> Review the sustainable development goals in *Figure 4.1*; how achievable do you think each one is?

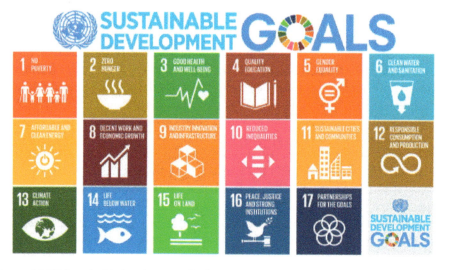

**Figure 4.1** *UN Sustainable Development Goals.*

> **ACTIVITY 4.3**
>
> Explore your country's public health policies. What are the priorities within your country? Do they match the SDGs? Are their priorities focused on future generations? For example, Wales has the Well-Being of Future Generations Act (Welsh Government, 2015) and a Future Generations Commissioner.

## 4.3 Epidemiology

Global public health policy and initiatives are underpinned by data received from individual nations. This data (information) is epidemiological and allows health to be measured. Epidemiology is viewed as the *"foundation of public health"* (Detels, 2015, p. 403) as without it, diseases/conditions and health outcomes would be treated very differently and less effectively. It is the science behind public health practice and is essential in the prevention of health issues, promoting health and enhancing wellbeing. It allows us to understand patterns of diseases, their treatment and how the health of people can be improved. Epidemiology will be explored in this section of the chapter.

### 4.3.1 What is epidemiology?

Epidemiology is a way of exploring health and how, why and to whom disease presents. We often wonder why certain diseases occur within certain areas, within certain populations and if treatment is effective or not. All of these questions are researched and the findings (data) aid organisations in targeting pockets of disease prevalence in certain populations, e.g. outbreaks of measles, Ebola, coronavirus and flu. By understanding where, how and to whom a disease presents, appropriate treatment interventions can be established, implemented and evaluated. If necessary, changes may be made to the interventions based on evaluations, which will take the form of research findings. All of this activity sits within epidemiological studies and is a means to measuring health (Stewart, 2016).

The word epidemiology is a derivative of the Greek words *epi* (meaning 'on') and *demos* (meaning 'population'). Both words combined link to the word 'epidemic' (Saracci, 2010). An epidemic refers to the spread of a disease amongst populations. Epidemiology therefore is key when detecting such spread of disease and it has been used for thousands of years. There is historical data referring to the Greek physician Hippocrates (400 BC) which describes patterns of diseases such as tetanus and typhus. He recognised even then that health and disease were impacted on by what we would now call wider determinants of health; for example, the environment and certain lifestyle factors (Saracci, 2010).

Over the centuries, epidemiology has moved from observing and basing interventions on perception to a more insightful approach using data to analyse health status and disease prevalence in populations. Evidence is provided to instigate change which, in turn, can improve the population's health status. This occurred in 1854 in London when there was a cholera outbreak. Hundreds of people were dying and a doctor, named John Snow, started to collect information which included where people lived who were affected by cholera, as well as the facilities they had access to. Dr Snow found that that those affected by cholera lived very close to a particular water pump, which was subsequently found to be contaminated with raw sewage. Once a padlock was placed on the pump and the local population stopped using it, the number of recorded cases reduced. This is one of the earliest examples of epidemiology on record, where patterns of disease were explored which led to an intervention that was, in turn, evaluated for its impact (Saracci, 2010; Eliasz, 2019).

In the 21st century the role of epidemiology is still to explore, analyse and review patterns of disease. This allows an improved understanding of disease trends and their cause. Of course, epidemiology has evolved over time with advanced use of technology, resources and evidence-based knowledge.

> **ACTIVITY 4.4**
>
> Consider a recent public health issue – the re-emergence of measles. Think about how this was discovered.
> - How was the increase in cases detected?
> - Where were the most cases of measles?
> - Who reported the cases?
> - Who was most affected?
> - What were the public health measures put in place?

Epidemiology relates directly to nursing practice because it gives us answers that are relevant to our everyday work, for example: How common is the disease? Where is it occurring? Whom is it affecting? What needs to be done? The answers to these questions will require epidemiological data and can be applied to any infectious disease or long-term condition. You will see this sort of information used every day in healthcare practice and within evidence-based care. In relation to your answers to the questions in *Activity 4.4*, evidence suggests that the recent measles outbreak was due to the poor uptake of the measles, mumps and rubella (MMR) vaccine in the early 1990s. All of these illnesses are 'notifiable' which means that when an infectious disease is diagnosed it has to be reported to the public health department. The public health departments send this information to the Department of Health and Social Care, where they store this information, study it and feed it into the WHO. Weekly information for 2019 is accessible at bit.ly/PHW4-3-1.

Local information regarding infectious diseases triggers a response. Those most affected by the measles outbreak were young adults born in the 1990s and children whose parents were fearful of allowing their children to receive the MMR vaccine. The fear around the MMR vaccination related to the then doctor, Andrew Wakefield, erroneously linking the vaccine to autism. His research was entirely inaccurate and flawed to the extent that he was struck off the General Medical Council register. But the attention the findings of his research received panicked the general public and subsequently the uptake of the vaccination has decreased over recent years, and many countries have lost their 'measles-free' status. The trend in the rise of measles cases is a worldwide issue and local reports are indicating a current rise in mumps cases across the UK. Nationally and internationally, we would not know that we have an issue with measles if we did not gather and study epidemiological data. As you will explore in *Chapter 6*, public health measures are likely to be far-reaching. These may include the launch of targeted campaigns to improve the uptake of vaccines and an increase of immunisation clinics targeting teenagers and college/university students.

> **ACTIVITY 4.5**
>
> Reflect on how we measure health using epidemiology. Write a list of the different ways in which we collect data.

## 4.4 Genomics

Another way to detect abnormalities and screen populations to measure health status is the science of genomics. This section of the chapter provides an outline of genomics and considers its relevance in public health.

### 4.4.1 Definitions

Genomics is the study of people's deoxyribonucleic acid (DNA), whereas genetics studies certain genes. Sometimes these terms are interchanged but as explained below, they mean something different. Our bodies are made up of trillions of cells. Each cell has a core and this is called its nucleus; within the nucleus there are chromosomes which contain the DNA, as seen in *Figure 4.2*. DNA holds a special genetic code and has been described as the "recipe book" of the human body, because it stores so much information about the various types of protein within the DNA which makes it up, and holds all of our genetic information (HEE, 2017).

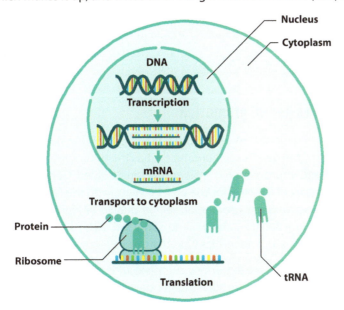

**Figure 4.2** *Cellular location of DNA and the processes of transcription and translation.*

All living organisms have a genome: animals, plants, bacteria and viruses. A genome is an organism's complete set of DNA, including all of its genes. Each genome contains all of the information needed to build and maintain that organism (Genomics England, 2020). DNA is made up of the molecules adenine (A), thymine (T), cytosine (C) and guanine (G) (U.S. National Library of Medicine, 2020), as indicated in *Figure 4.3*. There are billions of these chemicals in the human genome. They hold a wealth of information for researchers and are studied in genomic sequencing. This is where scientists use advanced technology that allows the removal of DNA for analysis and comparison with that of others, including close relatives, in order to determine whether there are any health concerns.

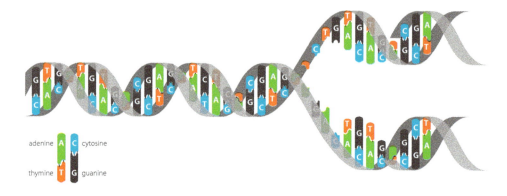

**Figure 4.3** *DNA structure.*

### ACTIVITY 4.6

Look up the following resources online:
- **Genomics England** bit.ly/4-6A
- **U.S. National Library of Medicine** bit.ly/4-6B
- **The Genomics Education Programme, Health Education England** bit.ly/4-6C
- **Genes and Health** bit.ly/4-6D
- **'From DNA to protein – 3D'** bit.ly/4-6E

## 4.4.2 Application to health promotion

So why is the study of genomes relevant within healthcare? What is so important about it? The study of the genome – 'genomics' – has the potential to predict disease, prevent it and improve how it is diagnosed and treated. Genetics with genomics has been part of the NHS for the past 70 years, with the first genetic counselling clinic set up in Great Ormond Street Hospital in 1946, some two years before the NHS was launched (Health Education England, 2019). *Figure 4.4* depicts how the study of genetics and genomics has advanced over the last 70 years.

Genomes and their make-up are extremely complex, with every genome being different. Advances in genomics are allowing the development of treatment for

4.4 Genomics

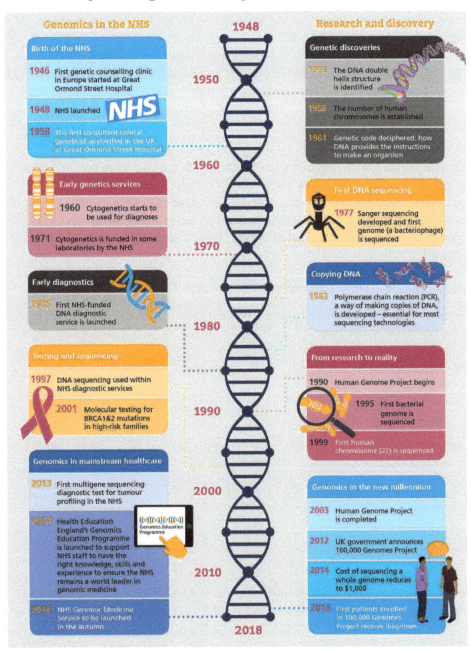

**Figure 4.4** History of genetics and genomics in healthcare.

patients which can prove preventative in the development of significant disease. In healthcare the 0.1% variation in the genome is of particular interest; 99% of our genomes are the same, and while some variations cause no problems, for example those which determine height, hair or eye colour, some can cause significant issues (HEE, 2017). Genomics can predict if someone will develop a genetic condition or if they are prone to a certain condition or disease. For example, some people have a particular gene mutation of the *BRCA1* or *BRCA2* gene which makes them at higher risk of developing breast cancer. *BRCA* stands for *BReast CAncer* gene. Based on this information, a risk assessment and special counselling inform those with the gene of their options. Some people proceed to undergo a double mastectomy (removal of both breasts). This decision is based on the information found in their genetic make-up via genetic testing. This has been given prominence in the media over recent years, with the actor Angelina Jolie undergoing this surgery.

The use of genomics in public health offers a preventative approach to healthcare. By determining the root cause of disease, through genome sequencing and genetic testing, specific treatment can be offered. To date, epidemiology has been responsive to emerging disease patterns and has focused on disease risk factors such as lifestyle choices or the environment. With the emergence of genomics, a more detailed picture can be obtained about the genetic make-up of individuals and an intervention can consider external influences as well as having a much more detailed picture of the disease. Genomics allows us to detect individuals who may inherit disease but also helps prevent progression of that disease. It is, therefore, a major public health breakthrough (Burton and Slade, 2017).

Genetic disorders may be single- or multifactorial gene inherited. Some single-gene inherited disorders include:

- cystic fibrosis
- Marfan syndrome
- Huntington's disease
- sickle cell anaemia
- fragile X syndrome.

Some multifactorial gene inherited disorders include:

- heart disease
- raised blood pressure
- Alzheimer's disease
- arthritis
- diabetes
- cancer
- obesity.

Genetic disorders can be diagnosed by genetic testing, which requires obtaining a sample of DNA. This can be collected in a number of ways, as a copy of our genome is in most of the cells in our bodies. DNA can be found in cells via blood, saliva, skin cells and hair roots, for example.

## 4.4.3 Application to public health

From a public health perspective, the advances in genomics will potentially have a significant impact on the health and wellbeing of populations. Genomic sequencing can help in the identification of an infection outbreak because bacteria are living organisms. They have a genome too with DNA, as humans do. So, by analysing their make-up and how they evolve, a specific treatment or intervention can be used to treat infection and diseases. The use of genomics can therefore aid in the control and treatment of certain infections, for example, TB or human immunodeficiency virus (HIV).

Genomics has also been key in examining antibiotic resistance. People are becoming resistant to certain antibiotics due to their overuse and changes within 'bacterial DNA'. These changes let the bacteria adapt and survive despite an antibiotic being administered. This can have a detrimental effect on patients and we have seen many outbreaks of methicillin-resistant *Staphylococcus aureus* (MRSA) which is very difficult to treat as it is resistant to certain antibiotics. Genomics is essential in investigating certain strains of bacteria, linking this to previous outbreaks and revealing the most appropriate antibiotic for these resistant infections. Some of the most common antibiotic-resistant infections are MRSA and penicillin-resistant *Enterococcus*. *Enterococcus* can cause endocarditis (inflammation of the lining of the heart), urinary tract infections, prostatitis (inflammation of the prostate gland), cellulitis and wound infections. Another well-known antibiotic resistant infection is multidrug-resistant *Mycobacterium tuberculosis* (MDR-TB). When antibiotic resistance occurs, this causes a major threat to recovery and can be life-threatening. In 2015 NICE introduced guidance around 'antimicrobial stewardship'. This guidance is aimed at health and social care professionals, organisations who fund and deliver care packages as well as the general public who take antimicrobials (antibiotics). Its aim is to avoid the overprescribing of antibiotics, as resistance to them is becoming a significant challenge within public health. It offers a set of good practice guidelines.

> **ACTIVITY 4.7**
>
> Explore the meaning of 'antimicrobial stewardship' in the NICE guideline NG15 *Antimicrobial stewardship: systems and processes for effective antimicrobial medicine use*, available at: www.nice.org.uk/guidance/ng15
>
> Consider how resistance to antibiotics is a threat to public health and identify what public health interventions are in place to prevent antibiotic resistance.

## 4.4.4 The role of the nurse in genomics

Health departments of the devolved administrations across the UK are promoting genomics to aid the detection, prevention and treatment of certain illnesses. Raising awareness of genomics will offer a greater knowledge base and understanding for healthcare staff which will, in turn, have a positive impact on patient care and health promotion/public health messages. This increased knowledge will allow the health professional to offer evidence-based health education advice with the aim of empowering individuals to partake in a healthier lifestyle. The advantages of this will include improved long-term health outcomes, reduced costs to healthcare services and, most importantly, improved health and wellbeing of patients (Calzone et al., 2018). Genomics within health education is now strongly recommended, with guidance on its inclusion in healthcare curricula along with frameworks for competence (Kirk, 2013; Kirk, Tonkin and Skirton, 2013).

### ACTIVITY 4.8

What is the nurse's role in genomics?

Nurses need to record a detailed family history concerning diseases, long-term conditions, ethnicity and information concerning lifestyle and cultural and religious beliefs from patients. They will also need to convey this information to appropriate healthcare professionals. In addition, Kirk, Tonkin and Skirton's (2013) revised framework of nursing competencies in genetics/genomics should be referred to. This is outlined below:

1. Clients need to be identified by completing an in-depth nursing assessment to determine if they would benefit from accessing genetic services.
2. Nurses need to be aware of the sensitive nature of genetic information and adapt information and services provided. This will depend on the client's culture, their knowledge base, language ability and developmental stage.
3. Nurses need to act as an advocate for their clients. This will allow informed decision-making.
4. Nurses need to have a knowledge and understanding of the role of genetics and genomics as well as how health is maintained and diseases prevented.
5. An awareness of the complex nature of genetic testing is required. This will allow evidence-based, competent care to be delivered to the client prior to, during and following any decision-making.
6. Practitioners need to reflect on and act on their own competency regularly, in relation to genetics knowledge.
7. Practitioners need to obtain and communicate credible, up-to-date contemporary information about genetics.
8. The provision of ongoing nursing care and support to patients, carers and families with genetic healthcare needs must be responsive in supporting any changing needs as they occur.

(Kirk, Tonkin and Skirton, 2013)

It is essential to work within your capabilities in relation to your involvement with patients undergoing any form of genetic testing. At whatever level you are practising, it is essential to have a basic knowledge of genomics and genetics to enhance clinical practice, especially from a public health perspective.

## 4.4.5 Preventative approaches to healthcare

There are a number of ways that disease prevention can be undertaken from a public health perspective. Screening is one approach and can be divided into primary, secondary and tertiary prevention. Although these approaches are well established, as outlined in *Chapter 2*, their scope is developing significantly because of developments in genomics. Primary prevention is linked to preventing a disease from occurring. Secondary prevention relates to early diagnosis and treatment, with the aim of stopping the progression of a disease through treatment or lifestyle change. Tertiary prevention is concerned with putting interventions in place to reduce the repercussions of a disease (Green *et al.*, 2015).

> **ACTIVITY 4.9**
>
> Identify some examples of screening from a primary, secondary and tertiary prevention perspective, based on the above definitions.

Some examples of primary prevention screening which are underpinned by genomics are shown below:
- Antenatal screening with the use of ultrasound scanning and/or blood tests can detect certain inherited conditions. Blood tests, for example, can detect sickle cell anaemia or thalassaemia, whereas ultrasound scanning can detect spina bifida. Mothers are screened for HIV and hepatitis B.
- A combination of blood tests and ultrasound scans can detect the likelihood of certain syndromes, such as Down syndrome.
- Neonatal screening can be carried out for conditions such as phenylketonuria, which is detected by newborn blood spot screening. This is a metabolic disorder which prevents the breakdown of the amino acid phenylalanine. This is a protein and in excess it causes significant brain damage. Therefore, earlier diagnosis and treatment (low-protein diet) offers a reduced risk of complications.

An example of secondary prevention screening is:
- familial raised cholesterol testing – if a person has raised cholesterol over 7.5mmol/L and a family history of raised cholesterol, DNA testing should be recommended (Burton and Slade, 2017). This allows for a treatment plan to be put in place, as well as lifestyle changes to reduce the risk of heart disease and stroke later on in life.

Examples of tertiary prevention screening include:
- breast cancer screening such as mammography post-diagnosis and family history.
- pathogen whole genome sequencing, which allows the detection of certain pathogens, such as MRSA. Once discovered, interventions can be put in place to eradicate or control the pathogen (Burton and Slade, 2017).

The above examples demonstrate how essential genomics is in the prevention of disease and protection of the general population worldwide. Epidemiological data, alongside the advancement of genome sequencing and genetic testing, has the potential to significantly improve health outcomes by allowing people to receive treatment earlier and to be provided with advice and support concerning changes to their lifestyles, if required.

## 4.5 Wider determinants of health

As a final point in this chapter, we need to revisit the issues raised in *Chapters 2* and *3* regarding the broader determinants of health beyond genomics, since these have a significant impact on lifestyle change, uptake of treatment and access to services.

As we have seen, the wider determinants of health, or social determinants of health as they are also known, are well documented. Dahlgren and Whitehead's (1991) rainbow model (see *Section 2.2*) demonstrates that individuals have their own unique factors that influence their health, and genetics play an important role in this. However, there are additional factors, as we have seen, that impact on an individual's or a community's health.

The aim of global public health is to ensure that individuals have access to relevant health services, education, clean water and sanitation, affordable and clean energy, are able to live free of poverty and have access to work. These are just some of the sustainable development goals referred to in *Section 4.2* and seen in *Figure 4.1*. In *Case study 4.1* we can see how genomics, the wider determinants of health and global health priorities come together to influence an individual's health.

### CASE STUDY 4.1 BETH

Beth, aged 35, is the mother of two children, a girl aged 5 and a boy aged 3. She has access to social housing and lives in a two-bedroomed semi-detached new build on the outskirts of a city in the UK. Beth has some support from her family, particularly her mum, who is her main support. Her mum is recovering from breast cancer and, following a mastectomy last year, is making good progress. Beth has a sister, aged 30, who works away and a brother, aged 25, who is travelling. Beth is in an on/off relationship with her partner. Their relationship is quite volatile at times but Beth won't tolerate shouting around the children. Beth is well educated and has a degree in sociology which she has never really used. Her work experience is mainly bar work with some singing experience. She works an odd shift in her local pub, but this is sporadic. She accesses the benefits she is eligible to, but this barely meets her weekly outgoings. She is currently looking for a job, but she would really like to train to become a midwife. Beth smokes about 10 cigarettes a day and is trying to quit.

## ACTIVITY 4.10

Reflecting on the previous components of this chapter, consider the following:
- How is Beth affected by the social determinants of health?
- What influences her lifestyle choices?
- How could Beth make healthier choices?
- Do you have any concerns regarding her genetic history?
- What could Beth do to improve her situation?
- What support could she access from her local health services?

It appears that Beth has the potential to live a healthy life. From a social determinants perspective, she is struggling financially, has potential childcare issues and the impact of her volatile relationship may hamper access to support. In responding to *Activity 4.10* you may have considered the outer aspects of Dahlgren and Whitehead's (1991) model, which address general socioeconomic, cultural and environmental conditions. These are macro issues that are influenced by policy makers, governments and public health departments. Although Beth may feel that she has little influence on these factors, her demographic information would contribute to epidemiological data which will, in turn, inform policy. For example, she is unemployed, receiving benefits and smokes. The UN's (UN General Assembly, 2015) seventeen SDGs will also contribute to policy development at the national level. While these goals and national policy seem removed from some members of society, they are influenced somewhat from the bottom up, by local areas providing demographic information to public health departments. Epidemiological data also influences this.

In relation to genomics, Beth's mum has had breast cancer. You may have considered the potential impact for Beth, whether there is a genetic link and whether Beth will have access to specialist services to screen her. All of this information about individuals informs public health practice.

The social determinants of health can have a detrimental impact on the uptake of services. Health services are influenced by healthy public policy (see *Chapter 6*) but also have to be focused on the individual's need and health status. Health needs and status vary enormously across the world. Individuals need resources to change their behaviours but access to services is not always possible due to a wide range of barriers such as financial issues, transport, housing and poor general health. The wider determinants of health, therefore, need careful consideration within any health promotion intervention. Many individuals live in complex situations affected by their individual sociopolitical contexts and health inequalities. This can affect their psychological as well as their physical wellbeing and can have a detrimental effect on motivation to pursue a healthier life course. Nurses are in a prime position to support, educate and empower individuals and, therefore, influence population health, while considering the impact of the wider determinants of health.

## KEY LEARNING POINTS

Four key points to take away from *Chapter 4*:
- ☑ The sustainable development goals set the context and act as drivers for global public health with a major focus on climate change, reducing health inequality and eradicating poverty. These global drivers underpin national policy in an attempt to improve the health and wellbeing of future generations.
- ☑ Epidemiology is the foundation of public health and aids the investigation of the health status of populations by examining disease prevalence, treatment and intervention.
- ☑ Genomics, genome sequencing and genetic testing will potentially improve health outcomes, allowing people to receive treatment earlier and to be supported in making changes to their lifestyles, if required.
- ☑ The wider determinants of health can have a significant impact on lifestyle change, the uptake of treatment and access to services and must be considered in all interventions.

# REFERENCES

Abdalla, S. and Ognenis, S. (2019) 'Key concepts in global health'. In Sethia, B. and Kumar, P. (eds) *Essentials of Global Health*. Elsevier.

Burton, H. and Slade, I. (2017) *Public Health and Genomics*. Genomics in mainstream medicine. PHG Foundation.

Calzone, K., Kirk, M., Tonkin, E. *et al.* (2018) Increasing nursing capacity in genomics: overview of existing global genomics resources. *Nurse Education Today,* **(69):** 53–59.

Dahlgren, G. and Whitehead, M. (1991) *Policies and Strategies to Promote Social Equity in Health*. Stockholm Institute for Futures Studies.

Detels, R. (2015) 'Epidemiology: the foundation of public health'. In Detels, R., Gulliford, M., Karim, Q. and Tan, C. (eds) *Oxford Textbook of Global Public Health*, 6th edition. Oxford University Press.

Eliasz, M. (2019) 'A history of global health'. In Sethia, B. and Kumar, P. (eds) *Essentials of Global Health*. Elsevier.

Genomics England (2020) *What is a genome?* Available at: www.genomicsengland.co.uk/understanding-genomics/what-is-a-genome/ (accessed 12 May 2020)

Green, J., Tones, K., Cross, R. and Woodall, J. (2015) *Health Promotion: planning and strategies*. SAGE.

Health Education England (2017) *Genomics Education Programme*. The Genomics game, midwifery version. HEE/NHS/Focus Games.

Health Education England (2019) *70 Years of Genetics and Genomics in Healthcare*. Available at: www.genomicseducation.hee.nhs.uk/blog/70-years-of-genetics-and-genomics-in-healthcare/ (accessed 12 May 2020)

Kirk, M. (2013) Introduction to genetics and genomics: a revised framework for nurses. *Nursing Standard,* **28(8):** 37–41.

Kirk, M., Tonkin, E. and Skirton, H. (2013) An iterative consensus-building approach to revising a genetics/genomics competency framework for nurse education in the UK. *Journal of Advanced Nursing,* **70(2):** 405–20.

Saracci, R. (2010) *Epidemiology: a very short introduction*. Oxford University Press.

Sethia, B. and Kumar, P. (eds) (2019) *Essentials of Global Health*. Elsevier.

Stewart, A. (2016) *Basic Statistics and Epidemiology: a practical guide*, 4th edition. Taylor and Francis.

UN General Assembly (2015) *Transforming our World: the 2030 agenda for sustainable development*. Available at: https://sustainabledevelopment.un.org/content/documents/21252030%20Agenda%20for%20Sustainable%20Development%20web.pdf (accessed 12 May 2020)

UN (2019) *Sustainable Development Goals*. Available at: https://www.un.org/sustainabledevelopment/development-agenda/ (accessed 12 May 2020)

U.S. National Library of Medicine (2020) *What is DNA?* Available at: www.ghr.nlm.nih.gov/primer/basics/dna (accessed 12 May 2020)

Welsh Government (2015) Well-Being of Future Generations (Wales) Act 2015. Welsh Government.

# Chapter 5
# Enabling, mediating and advocating in health promotion

Clare Bennett, Sue Lillyman and Katharine Whittingham

**LEARNING OUTCOMES**

When you have finished this chapter you should be able to:

5.1 Apply the terms enabling, mediating and advocating to health promotion

5.2 Discuss the relevance of the social gradient of health across the life course

5.3 Demonstrate an understanding of the key issues affecting the health of children, young people, older people, families, women and men

5.4 Outline the significance of health inequalities on lifestyle

5.5 Explore how health services address health promotion across the life course.

## 5.1 Introduction

As we have seen in the previous chapters, the WHO's Ottawa Charter for Health Promotion (WHO, 1986) remains central to our approach to health promotion. This chapter focuses on the WHO's three basic strategies for health promotion: enabling, mediating and advocacy, which are required for all health promotion action areas. In order to make these strategies meaningful, we will examine them in the context of the lifespan with a focus on the different needs of men, women, children, young people, families and older people, in relation to inequalities within and across these groups.

## 5.2 Defining enabling, mediating and advocating

*Figure 5.1* is the WHO's (1986) health promotion emblem. The logo incorporates five key action areas in health promotion:
- build healthy public policy
- create supportive environments for health
- strengthen community action for health
- develop personal skills

*Chapter 5: Enabling, mediating and advocating in health promotion*

- re-orientate health services.

These action areas are at the heart of the subsequent chapters of this book. The outer circle depicts the goal of building *"healthy public policies"* and emphasises that policy is pivotal to stability and coherence. The circle encompasses three wings, which aim to convey the message that all five key action areas need to be addressed. The small circle represents the three basic strategies for health promotion: enabling, mediating and advocacy. These apply to each health promotion action area. The aim of the logo is to emphasise that health promotion can only have impact through comprehensive, multi-strategy, integrated designs.

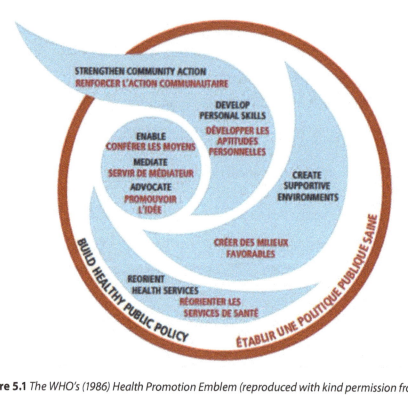

**Figure 5.1** *The WHO's (1986) Health Promotion Emblem (reproduced with kind permission from WHO:* www.who.int/healthpromotion/conferences/previous/ottawa/en/index4.html) *The Ottawa Charter for Health Promotion First International Conference on Health Promotion, Ottawa, 21 November 1986).*

## 5.2.1 Enabling

In the context of health promotion, the WHO (1998) states that enabling refers to professionals, such as nurses,

> ... *taking action in partnership with individuals or groups to empower them, through the mobilization of human and material resources, to promote and protect their health.*

(WHO, 1998, p. 7)

*5.2 Defining enabling, mediating and advocating*

The definition's emphasis on empowerment through partnership and on the mobilisation of resources demonstrates the important role nurses can play in this aspect of health promotion strategy development and implementation. Nurses have a vital role in providing populations and individuals with access to information on health and by facilitating skills development in communities and individuals. A further approach that nurses can use to enable individuals and groups of people is to support them in accessing the political processes which shape public policies affecting health.

> **ACTIVITY 5.1**
>
> Identify instances where you have seen enabling in action. What actions did the nurse take and what were the outcomes?

It is likely that you will have observed enabling in a variety of guises. In the UK, enabling is commonly seen in the management of long-term conditions, where the nurse supports a patient in developing the necessary skills to self-manage their condition. In the field of sexual health promotion, examples may include nurses supporting patients with genital herpes to enhance their health-related quality of life through relaxation techniques (since stress is related to recurrences) and the self-administration of oral suppressive antiviral therapies when they have a recurrence. Another example, aimed at primary prevention, may involve nurses working with young people to help them recognise indicators of coercive control and actions to take if they recognise that they are in an abusive relationship, or negotiation skills to enable young people to negotiate the kind of relationships they want, which may include safe sex. In relation to mobilising resources, nurses are commonly involved in providing condoms and contraception across the lifespan.

> **ACTIVITY 5.2**
>
> Access the Royal College of Nursing's Domestic Abuse Pocket Guide at bit.ly/A5-2
>
> How could you use this information to "enable" patients in your care?

## 5.2.2 Mediating

In health promotion, mediation is:

> … *a process through which the different interests (personal, social, economic) of individuals and communities, and different sectors (public and private) are reconciled in ways that promote and protect health.*
>
> (WHO, 1998, p. 16)

In health promotion, we often discuss 'health promotion settings'. Such settings may include healthy cities, schools, hospitals and universities, amongst others. As you can imagine, trying to meet the needs of all parties in such settings will require much mediation. Dooris *et al.* (2012) give the example of developing healthy universities, highlighting the challenges that can occur in introducing and integrating a commitment to health in a sector that does not hold health as a central aim. They argue that mediation has to clearly demonstrate why the university is such an important setting for health promotion and that investment in the health of students, staff and the local community can positively impact upon the university's core business; for example, through enhancing student and staff recruitment, retention, achievement and productivity. At this point in your career you may imagine that such discussions have little relevance to nursing, but nurses in public health roles are often key to such mediation. For example, an occupational health nurse may mediate with commercial companies to provide safe working environments for employees such as protective equipment, or a public health nurse may mediate with schools regarding the availability of hand-washing facilities.

> **ACTIVITY 5.3**
>
> Visit www.ted.com, search for and watch "William Ury: the walk from 'no' to 'yes'". Consider how you could use Ury's guidance about mediation in your practice as a nurse.

### 5.2.3 Advocating

Advocacy for health is:

> … *a combination of individual and social actions designed to gain political commitment, policy support, social acceptance and systems support for a particular health goal or programme.*
>
> (WHO, 1998, p. 5)

Advocacy may take many forms, including the use of the mass media, multimedia and political lobbying. It may also take the form of community mobilisation, as we will see in *Chapter 8*. Nurses have a significant responsibility to advocate for health at all levels in society. A recent example of a nurse demonstrating an advocacy role in health promotion relates to Claire Murdoch's letter to five major gambling companies. At the time of writing Claire Murdoch was NHS England's National Mental Health Director and had been a registered mental health nurse for 34 years. An example of one of the letters is provided in *Figure 5.2*.

Other high-profile advocacy roles that healthcare professionals are currently involved in concern the removal of harmful images, such as self-harm, from social media platforms. However, the nurse's role in advocacy can also be less high profile. For example, an allergy nurse specialist may advocate for a child with peanut allergy in making school a safe place by making it nut-free. As you may be thinking, this is likely to require mediation too, since this would require a concerted effort on the part of the school.

In practice, the three basic strategies for health promotion (enabling, mediating and advocacy) are often used simultaneously in order to support individuals and populations in promoting their health. We will now apply these strategies in the context of the lifespan with a focus on the different needs of women, men, young people, families and older people in relation to inequalities within and across these groups.

Dear Ms ▇▇▇ and Mr ▇▇▇,

I am writing regarding the increasingly clear and worrying links between gambling and mental ill health.

As the head of England's mental health services and a nurse of more than 30 years' experience, I have seen first-hand the devastating impact on mental wellbeing of addiction and am concerned that the prevalence of gambling in our society is causing harm.

In particular, the reports of certain tactics used by firms to target those of your customers who have already lost sums and are willing to bet more, to seek to recover losses are concerning.

If reports are correct I am concerned that offering people who are losing vast sums of money free tickets, VIP experiences, and free bets, all proactively prompt people back into the vicious gambling cycle which many want to escape.

You will know that in response to the fact that 430,000 people now have a serious betting problem, the NHS is opening gambling addiction clinics across the country.

For seven decades the NHS has adapted services in response to current challenges, but we should not be expected to pick up the pieces from lives damaged by avoidable harm.

In order to operate safely, the gambling industry has a responsibility to prevent the occasional flutter turning into a dangerous habit.

Worryingly some of the incentives apparently offered by individual firms to continue betting, appear designed to undermine people's ability to stay in control: bet to view streaming; pervasive advertising; and rewards in exchange for bets, all are likely to make decision-making for vulnerable people significantly harder.

As such, I am requesting that you please provide urgent detail on actions that your firm – and the industry – is taking to reduce the likelihood and severity of gambling addiction.

An industry-wide effort is needed to tackle this, and I am seeking reassurance that your organisation is taking measures, including the following, to minimise harm:

- Immediately ban credit card bets from your websites – ahead of the gambling commission's restrictions due to come into force later this year - helping ensure people don't spend money they don't have and potentially rack up life changing debt and the anxiety that comes with it;
- Stop the targeting of high-loss customers with the so-called 'VIP' treatment which includes incentives such as free tickets and bets;
- End bet to view commercial deals which require a stake in exchange for sports streaming access.

I look forward to your response.

**Figure 5.2** *Example of a letter to a gambling company from NHS England. Adapted from* Links between gambling and mental ill health: letters from Claire Murdoch.

## 5.3 A life-course approach to health promotion

PHE (2019) and WHO (2018) promote a life-course approach to the prevention of ill health (primary prevention) and the relevance of the life course to health outcomes is emphasised by Marmot (2020). PHE (2019) summarises positive and negative influences across the life course as detailed in *Table 5.1*.

**Table 5.1** *Positive and negative influences across the life course (PHE, 2019)*

| Protective factors | Risk factors |
| --- | --- |
| A healthy balanced diet | Smoking |
| An environment that enables physical activity | Adverse childhood experiences |
| Good educational attainment | Crime and violence |
| Being in stable employment with a good income | Drug and alcohol misuse |
| Living in good quality housing | Poor educational attainment |
| Having networks of support, including friends and family | Poor mental health |

PHE (2019) argues that if we address the wider determinants of health, people's health status and wellbeing can be significantly enhanced. They, therefore, promote a life-course approach to health promotion and outline what they describe as "critical stages in life" where positive differences can be made to the health and wellbeing of individuals and populations. The life stages are:

- Preconception
- Infancy and early years (0–5 years)
- Childhood and adolescence (5–24 years)
- Working age and adults (16–64 years)
- Older people.

Good functional ability is a key goal of the life-course approach. Functional ability refers to an individual's *"capacity to carry out the activities that he or she needs or wishes to carry out in a given environment"* (Lehto et al., 2017, p. 15). Supportive environments, facilitated by health policy, the environment and social norms are pivotal in ensuring that individuals can maximise their functional ability. An example of this in action is the creation of dementia-friendly towns and communities which prioritise the availability of dementia-friendly accommodation, social opportunities, transport, pathways, signage and lighting. By creating an environment that supports people living with dementia in socialising and optimising their independence, the individual's functional ability is enhanced. There are many examples of such communities throughout the UK which you can easily find if you use the search terms 'dementia friendly communities' online.

The following discussions will consider specific life-course approaches to health promotion.

## 5.3.1 Preconception and becoming a parent

Interventions during the preconception period and pregnancy can significantly influence physical, cognitive and emotional outcomes for the child both during childhood and subsequently. If a pregnancy is planned, the preconception period presents nurses with the opportunity to promote healthy behaviours amongst prospective parents, including:

- health screening
- assessment of genetic conditions including sickle cell and thalassaemia
- establishing vaccination status pre-pregnancy, e.g. MMR vaccinations
- taking folic acid supplements
- healthy diet
- being physically active
- smoking cessation
- reducing alcohol consumption (PHE, 2019).

For more detailed information access the *Health Matters* resource on reproductive health and pregnancy planning at bit.ly/S5-3-1.

> ### ACTIVITY 5.4
>
> Enabling smoking cessation is an integral part of the nurse's role in health promotion and when it is in the context of pregnancy, the nurse also has an advocacy role in relation to the unborn child. Access NICE's Stop Smoking Guidelines at www.nice.org.uk/guidance/ng92 to appraise yourself of the most up-to-date resources and approaches available.

## 5.3.2 Infancy and early years (0–5 years)

PHE (2016) emphasises the importance of the first 1000 days of a child's life in relation to their subsequent health and wellbeing. Marmot (2020) also emphasises the critical impact that early childhood experiences can have on health outcomes. Parenting style, socioeconomic status and the quality of early education and care significantly impact upon a child's cognitive development and health, as well as their mental wellbeing and socioeconomic status in adulthood.

The development of communication skills in young children is pivotal and early language is a primary indicator of child wellbeing. The Healthy Child Programme (Asmussen and Brims, 2018), which is available at bit.ly/S5-3-2, is an evidence-based framework for universal prevention and early intervention. The programme is concerned with child health promotion, child health surveillance, screening, immunisations, child development reviews, prevention and early intervention to improve outcomes for children and reduce inequalities. The majority of the programme is supported by health visitors, family health nurses and nurses working in primary care.

> **ACTIVITY 5.5**
>
> PHE (2019) states that:
>
> > After clean water, vaccination is the most effective public health intervention in the world for saving lives and promoting good health. The UK has one of the best immunisation programmes in the world and recently introduced the world's first infant meningitis B vaccination programme.
>
> Throughout the UK there is a strong anti-vaccination movement, but in your role as a nurse it is essential to advocate for childhood immunisations. Use the internet to explore the arguments of anti-vaccine groups and compare these with the evidence presented at bit.ly/A5-5.

### 5.3.3 Childhood and adolescence (5–24 years)

Throughout childhood and adolescence, children and young people are likely to engage in risky behaviour, although the degree to which they engage in high-risk behaviours will be shaped by peer pressure, social media, family and the wider community (Department of Health and Social Care and PHE, 2018). PHE's (2018a) report *School aged years high impact area 2: Keeping safe: Reducing risky behaviours. School nurses leading the Healthy Child Programme 5–19* emphasises the important role that school nurses can play in enabling children to become confident, healthy adults. Some of the key issues that face this age group are addressed below.

**Safeguarding**

The Crime Survey for England and Wales (CSEW) estimated that one in five adults aged 18 to 74 years experienced at least one form of child abuse, such as emotional abuse, physical abuse, sexual abuse, or witnessed domestic violence or abuse, before the age of 16 years (ONS, 2020). Around half of adults (52%) who experienced abuse before the age of 16 years also experienced domestic abuse later in life, compared with 13% of those who did not experience abuse before the age of 16 years (ONS, 2020).

Many cases of abuse remain hidden and the Department for Education (2018) emphasises the need for a child-centred approach to safeguarding which involves all practitioners that come into contact with children and young people taking appropriate action. Enabling, advocating and mediating are all relevant to this aspect of the nurse's role. A child or young person cannot flourish and achieve their full functional ability if they are exposed to:

- physical and emotional abuse
- neglect
- exploitation by criminal gangs and organised crime groups
- trafficking
- online abuse
- sexual exploitation
- the influences of extremism leading to radicalisation.

Regardless of the nature of abuse or neglect, nurses must put the needs of children first when determining what action to take. A particularly challenging aspect of safeguarding relates to female genital mutilation (FGM). FGM, sometimes known as female circumcision or female genital cutting, involves the removal of part or all of the external genitalia of women and girls using a sharp object such as a knife, scalpel, scissors, glass or razor blade. Such instruments are often unsterilised and anaesthesia is rarely used, with girls and women often being subject to forceful restraint (NSPCC, 2019).

It is estimated that 10 000 girls born overseas and now living in England and Wales have experienced FGM (PHE, 2018a). FGM is a very complex issue because of its associated cultural beliefs. However, FGM is illegal in the UK and it is also illegal to take a British national or permanent resident abroad for FGM. A number of campaigns have been successful in enabling young women to seek support if they feel that they are at risk of FGM. One campaign, which originated in Gothenburg, is the 'hide a spoon in your knickers' campaign, which is promoted to girls who feel that they are being taken abroad for a forced marriage or FGM. The presence of a spoon will trigger metal detectors at airport security and staff in airports are trained to support potential victims. This initiative has been widely disseminated throughout the UK.

> **ACTIVITY 5.6**
>
> Look up the RCN's guidance concerning FGM at bit.ly/5-6A.
>
> Healthcare professionals are required by law to alert the police if they treat a girl under 18 who has had FGM. This professional duty is a mandatory requirement for all nurses. It is a personal duty; it cannot be transferred to anyone else.
> - Seek guidance from your Health Board or Trust as to what mechanisms you should follow to report FGM.
> - Identify enabling, mediating and advocating strategies that are relevant to nurses in the context of FGM and discuss these with senior nurses in your clinical area to see how they are enacted in practice.

**Tobacco, alcohol and drug use**

PHE (2018b) has identified that children and young people who are disadvantaged are more likely to smoke and engage in drug use. This is particularly the case amongst young offenders, those not in education, employment or training (NEET), truants, care leavers, the homeless or those living in socioeconomically disadvantaged areas.

Two-thirds of smokers start to smoke before the age of 18 (PHE, 2019). Reasons are complex and include peer pressure, experimentation and behavioural problems. Children are more likely to smoke if they live with others who smoke. Smoking cessation aimed at parents and carers can, therefore, be health-promoting for children and young people.

### Sexual health

Unintended teenage pregnancies and sexually transmitted infections can have adverse physical, psychological and social consequences for young people. Nurses can play a key role in enabling young people to enhance their sexual health by lobbying for services that are accessible for young people through their role as advocates, by mediating with settings that young people access to ensure that sexual health promotion is available as well as through direct activities that empower young people to assert themselves in relationships. Furthermore, nurses are central to the human papillomavirus (HPV) vaccination programme which is offered to all school pupils, both male and female, aged 12 and 13 years, to protect against cervical, oral, throat and anal cancers.

#### ACTIVITY 5.7

Access *Sexual and Reproductive Health and HIV: applying All Our Health* at bit.ly/A5-7
- List the consequences of poor sexual health for individuals
- Access the sexual and reproductive health and HIV e-learning session
- Consider how you can enable, advocate and mediate in order to promote the sexual health of an individual and/or community

## 5.3.4 Working age and adults (16–64 years)

### Men's health

Gender equality is a fundamental human right and is reflected in the UN's SDG 3, to *"ensure healthy lives and promote well-being for all"* (WHO, 2016). However, we know that men globally have a lower life expectancy than women; for example, the WHO statistics for 2019 predicted that boys born in 2018 could expect to live an average of 68.6 years and girls 73.1 years.

#### ACTIVITY 5.8

Make a list of the reasons why men have a reduced life expectancy.

Many of the items on your list are likely to relate to men's lifestyle behaviours. These, according to Ragonese, Shand and Barker (2019), include seven key health behaviours:
- poor diet
- tobacco use
- alcohol use
- occupational hazards
- unsafe sex
- drug use
- limited health-seeking behaviour.

Purnell (2019) adds to this list by highlighting risk-taking behaviours amongst men, especially those under the age of 25 years, with mortality being most likely to be related to violence and road traffic accidents. Suicide has also been reported as the highest single cause of death for men aged under 50 years, in the UK (Mental Health Foundation, 2019). Additional factors, as we saw in *Chapter 3*, relate to health-seeking behaviours and occupational hazards are also greater in men than women since men tend to have more roles in construction, driving, mining and the military.

In addressing the specific health promotion needs of men, one of the first areas we need to identify is the strong beliefs, norms, attitudes and stereotypes of masculinity. Ragonese, Shand and Barker (2019) note the need to change social norms that reinforce resultant behaviours such as self-sufficiency, stoicism, risk taking and hypersexuality. Advocating for an improvement in health literacy amongst men can help promote their health-seeking behaviours, in addition to providing gender-sensitive interventions that are aimed at men (Baker, 2016). It is interesting to note, however, that at the time of writing there are only four countries that have national health policies or strategies specially aimed at men: Ireland, Brazil, Iran and Australia (Ragonese, Shand and Barker, 2019).

> **ACTIVITY 5.9**
>
> Read the National Men's Health Action Plan Healthy Ireland – Men HI-M 2017–2021 Working with men in Ireland to achieve optimum health and wellbeing at bit.ly/5-9A
>
> In particular, review Appendix 5 as this includes some more detail in relation to the need for this action plan.

**Women's health**

The UN SDGs 2016–2030 aim to end world poverty, protect the planet and ensure prosperity (UN, 2016). Importantly for women's health, two of these goals focus on addressing the health needs of girls and women and include the following targets:

> … reduce the global maternal mortality ratio to less than 70 per 100,000 live births and to ensure universal access to sexual and reproductive health care services including contraceptive services, information and education.
>
> (UN, 2016)

The targets set out by the UN present a major public health challenge for health and social care providers when considering the evidence of inequalities for women's health across the lifespan. In 2010 the Marmot Review *Fair Society, Healthy Lives* (Marmot, 2010) demonstrated systemic gender differences in health outcomes. Marmot's (2020) more recent review highlighted how these inequalities have endured and, in some instances, widened over time. These aspects of women's health will now be discussed.

> **ACTIVITY 5.10**
>
> Make a list of the key determinants of women's health.

While women live longer than men, they experience a higher proportion of their lives in poor health. As you may have considered when addressing *Activity 5.10*, this poor health can be related to lifestyle behaviours including smoking, diet, alcohol intake and engagement with physical activity. While alcohol intake has declined over the last few years, 14% of women in the UK population still drink more than the recommended maximum of 14 units of alcohol a week (NHS Digital, 2018). 42% of women are not engaging in adequate physical activity for good health (PHE, 2019). The consequences of these lifestyle behaviours include cardiovascular disease and type 2 diabetes. Furthermore, a key risk factor for developing cancer in women is obesity. Evidence indicates that being overweight can increase the risk of developing breast, ovarian and uterine cancer (Woolnough, 2017). Cervical and breast screening programmes and the introduction of the HPV vaccination programme have shown positive outcomes in reducing cancer.

However, social determinants of health are reflected in many of the inequalities in women's health. Women from lower socioeconomic groups, minority ethnic groups, women with mental health issues and learning and physical disabilities, and lesbian and bisexual women are less likely to access screening, thus making the health divide greater (Public Health England, 2017).

> **ACTIVITY 5.11**
>
> Consider how you, as a nurse, can make health screening, such as cervical screening, more accessible to minority ethnic groups, women with mental health issues, learning and physical disabilities, and lesbian and bisexual women.

### 5.3.5 Older people

Our ageing population is a public health success. Having more older people in society benefits us in many ways; for example, older people contribute financially, socially and culturally to communities (PHE, 2019). However, as people age, they are more prone to frailty, dementia and other co-morbidities associated with ageing. PHE (2019) asserts that as life expectancy rises, we must promote the concept of productive healthy ageing. Key areas include access to occupation (this may be in the form of paid employment, voluntary work or hobbies), suitable housing and external environments in which people feel safe to engage in outdoor activities, as well as vaccinations against flu, pneumococcal infection and shingles. Functional ability can also be enhanced by reducing the risk factors for dementia: stop smoking, be more active, reduce alcohol consumption and eat healthily, address depression, prevent falls and prevent loneliness and isolation (PHE, 2019).

## ACTIVITY 5.12

Think about the older people within your community or family. How can we as nurses promote healthy living for this generation by keeping them engaged in society and feeling useful?

## 5.4 Equality and diversity

According to Petty (2020) in her web post:

> *equality means ensuring everyone in your setting has equal opportunities, regardless of their abilities, their background or their lifestyle and diversity means appreciating the differences between people and treating people's values, beliefs, cultures and lifestyles with respect.*
>
> (Petty, 2020, online)

With these definitions in mind there are many areas within health promotion where we need to advocate and mediate for people to ensure people are treated fairly, equally, with dignity and respect regardless of their lifestyles and backgrounds. We also need to remember that this can include the right to refuse treatment for whatever reason, as long as the patient has mental capacity.

There has been a move in healthcare services, particularly in relation to care for people with disabilities, away from the 'fix it' medical model to the social model. The latter model focuses more on social barriers such as the environment, attitudes and organisational responsibilities and works with people to achieve their goals and aspirations in partnership with them regardless of their disability (RCN, 2020).

This move still needs to be addressed for people who are excluded from mainstream society due to their culture, lifestyle, preferences and/or beliefs. We need to be mindful of how we can help people from different backgrounds connect, or reconnect, with communities, families and society. Mulé *et al.* (2009) also highlighted this problem for the LGBT community, where there still needs to be a shift from the illness focus such as HIV/AIDS to a broader health and wellness approach for this group.

In order to meet everyone's needs we need to develop a trusting relationship which involves listening carefully to what they want and not assuming that we know, or understand, their individual needs and wants. To help achieve this we can build a relationship and advocate for people as individuals with different needs and then help them to address their own health and wellbeing goals.

> **ACTIVITY 5.13**
>
> - Find and read your Health Board or Trust's local policies and guidance on anti-discriminatory practice.
> - Look around your clinical area from a patient's perspective and see if you can see any areas of practice that may be unwittingly putting prejudices into practice. For example, does your practice expect people to phone in for appointments (which could be very difficult for those with hearing impairment), are you using the right language for people, avoiding stereotyping and are people with dementia given extra time and support?

## 5.5 Bringing the themes together: bioecological systems theory

Bronfenbrenner (2004) asserts that who we are and the actions that we may take, are largely influenced by our external environment and that if we want to change behaviour we have to change environments (Bronfenbrenner, 1979). He created the model which is summarised in *Figure 5.3*. The model consists of five distinct yet inter-related systems:

1. **Microsystem:** includes the immediate surroundings of an individual (family, school, peer group, neighbourhood) and one's personal biological make-up
2. **Mesosystem:** composed of *connections* between one's immediate environments (e.g. between the home and school, family and peer group)
3. **Exosystem:** made up of external environmental settings which only indirectly affect development (e.g. parent's workplace)
4. **Macrosystem:** the larger cultural context (e.g. national economy, political culture) or societal norms that have an impact on children's development by setting expectations for parental and child behaviour
5. **Chronosystem:** the influence of time on each of the settings and interactions in the system. As children develop, different settings and systems will have differing effects and impact in different ways.

The individual, at the centre of the model, has certain innate characteristics which will impact upon their development, such as gender, genetics and co-morbidities. However, Bronfenbrenner (1979, 2004) asserts that the external environments listed above will also have a significant impact upon the individual's development. Since development is linked to socioeconomic status, this model is significant in demonstrating how systems that are external to the individual play a vital role in one's health outcomes. Each of Bronfenbrenner's systems is relevant to nursing and the WHO's (1986) three basic strategies for health promotion: enabling, mediating and advocacy, since nurses have influence and a presence within each of the systems. For example, we are involved at the individual level; we are present in the microsystem through our involvement in schools, health services and places of employment; we have influence over the welfare services, mass media and communities which contribute to the exosystem; and within the macrosystem we can shape the attitudes and ideologies of the culture.

## 5.5 Bringing the themes together: bioecological systems theory

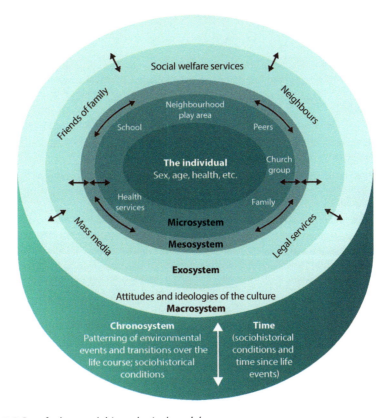

**Figure 5.3** *Bronfenbrenner's bioecological model.*

### ACTIVITY 5.14

Consider how Bronfenbrenner's bioecological model resonates with the various themes presented in this chapter: the nurse's role in enabling, mediating and advocating to facilitate health promotion, the social gradient of health, the life-course approach to health promotion and equality and diversity.

Consideration of this model is useful in highlighting how if we, as nurses, positively influence people's external environments, we can significantly enable people to promote their health and wellbeing.

### KEY LEARNING POINTS

Three key points to take away from *Chapter 5*:
- Enabling, mediating and advocating strategies are used simultaneously by nurses in order to promote health, both for the individual and within populations.
- Nurses are in a prime position to help people enhance their health and wellbeing across the lifespan.
- Health is often determined by the social gradient and age; however, nurses can assist in promoting health through advice on lifestyle choices and reducing risk-taking activities for all individuals.

# REFERENCES

Asmussen, K. and Brims, L. (2018) *What Works to Enhance the Effectiveness of the Healthy Child Programme: an evidence update.* Early Intervention Foundation. Available at: www.eif.org.uk/report/what-works-to-enhance-the-effectiveness-of-the-healthy-child-programme-an-evidence-update (accessed 13 May 2020).

Baker, P. (2016) Men's health: an overlooked inequality. *British Journal of Nursing*, **25(19)**: 1054–7.

Bronfenbrenner, U. (1979) *The Ecology of Human Development: experiments by nature and design.* Harvard University Press.

Bronfenbrenner, U. (2004) *Making Human Beings Human: bioecological perspectives on human development.* SAGE.

Department for Education (2018) *Working Together to Safeguard Children.* Available at: www.gov.uk/government/publications/working-together-to-safeguard-children--2 (accessed 13 May 2020)

Department of Health and Social Care and Public Health England (2018) School aged years high impact area 2: Keeping safe: Reducing risky behaviours. School nurses leading the Healthy Child Programme 5-19. Available at: https://assets.publishing.service.gov.uk/government/uploads/system/uploads/attachment_data/file/754803/school_aged_years_high_impact_area_2.pdf (accessed 13 May 2020)

Dooris, M., Doherty, S., Cawood, J. and Powell, S. (2012) 'The Healthy Universities approach: adding value to the higher education sector'. In Scriven, A. and Hodgins, M. (eds) *Health Promotion Settings: principles and practice.* SAGE.

Lehto, V., Jolanki, O., Valvanne, J., Seinelä, L. and Jylhä, M. (2017) Understanding functional ability: perspectives of nurses and older people living in long-term care. *Journal of Aging Studies*, **43**: 15–22. https://doi.org/10.1016/j.jaging.2017.09.001

Marmot, M. (2010) *Fair Society, Healthy Lives.* Available at: www.parliament.uk/documents/fair-society-healthy-lives-full-report.pdf (accessed 6 May 2020)

Marmot, M. (2020) *Health Equity in England: the Marmot Review 10 years on.* Institute of Health Equity. Available at: www.health.org.uk/sites/default/files/upload/publications/2020/Health%20Equity%20in%20England_The%20Marmot%20Review%2010%20Years%20On_full%20report.pdf (accessed 6 May 2020)

Mental Health Foundation (2019) *Mental Health Statistics: suicide.* Available at: www.mentalhealth.org.uk/statistics/mental-health-statistics-suicide (accessed 13 May 2020)

Mulé, N., Ross, L., Deeprose, B. *et al.* (2009) Promoting LGBT health and wellbeing through inclusive policy development. *Int J Equity Health*, **8(18)** DOI : org/10.1186/1475-9276-8-18

NHS Digital (2018) *Health Survey for England 2017.* Available at: https://digital.nhs.uk/data-and-information/publications/statistical/health-survey-for-england/2017 (accessed 13 May 2020)

NSPCC (2019) *Protecting Children from Female Genital Mutilation (FGM).* Available at: https://learning.nspcc.org.uk/child-abuse-and-neglect/fgm/ (accessed 13 May 2020)

Office for National Statistics (2020) *Child Abuse Extent and Nature, England and Wales: year ending March 2019.* Available at: www.ons.gov.uk/peoplepopulationandcommunity/crimeandjustice/articles/childabuseextentandnatureenglandandwales/yearendingmarch2019 (accessed 13 May 2020)

Petty, L. (2020) *How to Promote Equality & Diversity in Health & Social Care.* Available at: www.highspeedtraining.co.uk/hub/promoting-equality-diversity-health-social-care/ (accessed 13 May 2020)

Public Health England (2016) *Health Matters: giving every child the best start in life.* Available at: www.gov.uk/government/publications/health-matters-giving-every-child-the-best-start-in-life (accessed 13 May 2020)

Public Health England (2017) *NHS Screening Programmes*. Available at: https://assets.publishing.service.gov.uk/government/uploads/system/uploads/attachment_data/file/783537/NHS_Screening_Programmes_in_England_2017_to_2018_final.pdf (accessed 13 May 2020)

Public Health England (2018a) *School Aged Years High Impact Area 2: keeping safe: reducing risky behaviours. School nurses leading the Healthy Child Programme 5–19*. Available at: www.gov.uk/government/publications/commissioning-of-public-health-services-for-children (accessed 13 May 2020)

Public Health England (2018b) *Smoking, drinking and drug use among hard to reach children and young people; an evidence synthesis report*. Available at: www.basw.co.uk/system/files/resources/smoking_drinking_drug_use_among_hard_to_reach_children_and_young_people%20.pdf (accessed 13 May 2020)

Public Health England (2019) *Health Matters: prevention – a life course approach*. Available at: www.gov.uk/government/publications/health-matters-life-course-approach-to-prevention/health-matters-prevention-a-life-course-approach (accessed 13 May 2020)

Purnell, L. (2019) Men's health awareness. *Journal of Transcultural Nursing*, **30(6)**: 538–9.

Ragonese, C., Shand, T. and Barker, G. (2019) *Masculine Norms and Men's Health: making the connections*. Promundo-US. Available at: https://promundoglobal.org/wp-content/uploads/2019/02/Masculine-Norms-Mens-Health-Report_007_Web.pdf (accessed 13 May 2020)

Royal College of Nursing (2020) *The Social Model of Disability*. Available at: https://rcni.com/hosted-content/rcn/first-steps/social-model-of-disability (accessed 7 July 2020)

United Nations (2016) United Nations Sustainable Development Goals. Available at: www.undp.org/content/undp/en/home/sustainable-development-goals.html (accessed 13 May 2020)

Woolnough, S. (2017) *Cancer in Women: addressing unmet needs*. BMA. Available at: www.bma.org.uk/collective-voice/policy-and-research/public-and-population-health/womens-health (accessed 13 May 2020)

World Health Organization (1986) *Ottawa Charter for Health Promotion*. Available at: www.euro.who.int/__data/assets/pdf_file/0004/129532/Ottawa_Charter.pdf?ua=1 (accessed 6 May 2020)

World Health Organization (1998) *Health Promotion Glossary*. Available at: www.who.int/healthpromotion/about/HPG/en/ (accessed 13 May 2020)

World Health Organization (2016) *Sustainable Development Goal 3: ensure healthy lives and promote well-being for all at all ages*. Available at: https://sustainabledevelopment.un.org/sdg3 (accessed 13 May 2020)

World Health Organization (2018) *A Life-course Approach to Health: synergy with sustainable development goals*. Available at: http://dx.doi.org/10.2471/BLT.17.198358 (accessed 13 May 2020)

# Chapter 6
# Building a healthy public policy

Anneyce Knight

> **LEARNING OUTCOMES**
>
> When you have finished this chapter, you should be able to:
>
> **6.1** Define what healthy public policy is
>
> **6.2** Argue the requirement for the promotion of health to inform all policies and legislation
>
> **6.3** Describe the concept of a health needs analysis and what it may include
>
> **6.4** Outline what a health impact assessment is
>
> **6.5** Discuss key theories of how health literacy can be developed within populations.

## 6.1 Introduction

This chapter introduces you to some key concepts that contribute to building a healthy public policy in the UK. It includes an exploration of what healthy public policy is, the need for health promotion to be at the forefront of policy and legislation development, and discussion about Health Needs Analysis and Health Impact Assessment. A selection of theories related to developing health literacy are also outlined. As a society we need a healthy population, with individuals maintaining and enhancing their health throughout their lifespan, not only to ensure and enrich their quality of life but also, it is anticipated, to reduce NHS and social care expenditure.

## 6.2 Definitions and rationale

Your initial thoughts are probably, what is healthy public policy? We are very aware today that illness and disease have many contributing factors which are called the wider determinants of health. As we saw in *Chapters 2* and *4*, Dahlgren and Whitehead's (1991) rainbow model (*Figure 6.1*) illustrates these wider determinants. This diagram shows that individuals have their own unique factors that influence their health; for example, their genes, sex (gender) and age. Also, as you can see, the outer layers of the rainbow identify the wider factors (determinants) that can impact on the health of an individual or a community.

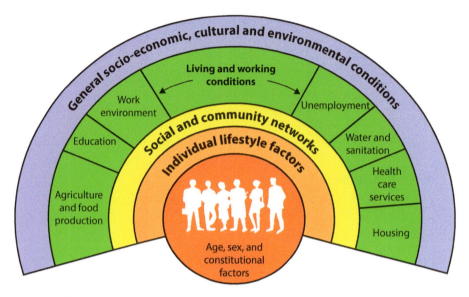

**Figure 6.1** *The Dahlgren–Whitehead rainbow. Reproduced by kind permission from: Dahlgren, G. and Whitehead, M. (1991) Policies and Strategies to Promote Social Equity in Health. Stockholm, Sweden: Institute for Futures Studies.*

### ACTIVITY 6.1

Think of one example for each of the social determinants specified below, from Dahlgren and Whitehead's model, which could have a negative impact on either an individual's health or your own health:
- Individual lifestyle
- Social and community networks
- General socioeconomic, cultural, environment

Public health addresses all the social determinants of health. As we saw in *Chapter 1*, the definition of public health used by the WHO is *"the art and science of preventing disease, prolonging life and promoting health through the organized efforts of society"* (Acheson, 1988). Public health is everybody's 'business' at individual, community, health and social care practitioner levels as well as local authority, national and international government policy-making level. Indeed, nationally each of the four UK nations strives to improve its population's public health and wellbeing and reduce health inequalities. Health inequalities are, for example, the difference in mortality rates between different socioeconomic groups or different geographical areas, as discussed in *Chapter 3*.

## ACTIVITY 6.2

Each of the four nations of the UK has a designated public health organisation which sets out its own country's strategies and priorities to improve health and wellbeing and reduce health inequalities.

Search the internet and find your nation's public health organisation (Public Health England, Public Health Scotland, Public Health Wales or Public Health Agency in Northern Ireland) and read about what its strategies and priorities are.

Overall, there are three overarching public health domains (FPH, 2016):
1. Health improvement, which aims to improve health behaviours and individual risk factors associated with poor health outcomes, which include the wider determinants of health.
2. Health protection, which ensures the provision of vaccination and immunisation programmes as well as assessing the health effects in relation to being exposed to factors such as biological or chemical agents, radiation or polluted water.
3. Healthcare public health which focuses on strategic development such as planning, procuring and monitoring healthcare services.

## ACTIVITY 6.3

- Identify two further individual lifestyle choices that people make that would put their health at risk, which are different from the one you identified in *Activity 6.1*.
- Note down an example of potential biological or chemical agents which may endanger the population.
- A local government travel plan and housing policy concludes that a local housing development of flats is to be built, specifically for vulnerable adults, next to the bus terminal. Consider the advantages and disadvantages in relation to health; for example, pollution, density of housing and access to amenities.

We can see that public health is very important and healthy public policy should reflect the need to improve and protect health with individual, family and community health promotion interventions. This needs to be alongside national legislation made by central government and each of the four nations' devolved governments. Furthermore, the concept of healthy public policy acknowledges that health is not solely the concern of each nation's NHS, as there are the wider social determinants of health.

The WHO Ottawa Charter of 1986 states:

> *Health promotion is the process of enabling people to increase control over, and to improve, their health. To reach a state of complete physical, mental and social well-being, an individual or group must be able to identify and to realize aspirations, to satisfy needs, and to change or cope with the environment. Health is, therefore, seen as a resource for everyday life, not the objective of living. Health is a positive concept emphasizing social and personal resources, as well as physical capacities. Therefore, health promotion is not just the responsibility of the health sector, but goes beyond healthy life-styles to well-being.*

(WHO, 1986)

So, healthy public policy aims to reduce health inequalities and *"to create a supportive environment to enable people to lead healthy lives"* (WHO, 1988). Examples include health promotion policies such as the Health Act of 2006 (HM Government, 2006) which meant that from 2007, in England, it was against the law to smoke in enclosed areas (for example workplaces, restaurants and pubs). (Note that all four UK nations have similar legislation in place.) It also includes other policy making that addresses wider social determinants of health, e.g. transport, housing, food standards, agriculture and health and safety.

## 6.3 Health in all policies

As we have seen, Dahlgren and Whitehead's model in *Section 6.1* shows that there are many influences on health. Although individuals can make personal choices that can improve their health (e.g. deciding to stop smoking, reducing their alcohol intake or eating their 5-a-day fruit and vegetables), many factors that impact on health are out of their direct control. For example, pollution, access to public transport, access to shops and health and safety at work are all dependent on local and national policies/legislation.

Health throughout the life course, 'from the cradle to the grave', is important so that everyone can fulfil their potential and achieve their dreams and aspirations whether in their education, their workplace or their retirement. It is imperative that local and national governments lead the way in ensuring that health and wellbeing inform all policy areas and that they are also aware of the impact these policies can have in maintaining and improving the health of communities.

Some examples of health and wellbeing being considered in policies and legislation are shown below.

Local government:
- plans to provide transport to villages to help minimise rural isolation.
- providing outdoor gyms, or trim trails, in local parks and green spaces, to provide free access for people to exercise.

### ACTIVITY 6.4

Think of a policy or legislation that the local government where you live could introduce to enhance the health of your local population.

National government:
- the Health Act 2006 (HM Government, 2006) banning smoking in public places (as noted previously)
- the Health and Safety at Work etc. Act 1974 (HM Government, 1974) which is the main legislation relating to occupational safety.

## 6.4 Assessing health needs

> **ACTIVITY 6.5**
>
> Think of a policy or legislation that the UK government could make to contribute to building a healthier population nationally.

Building a healthier population cannot be done based on policy and legislation development alone, as the wider determinants of health demonstrate. This requires collaborative and integrated working with the NHS, the public health departments and public health teams, the local authority and the voluntary sector working with local communities. In addition, empowering individuals and families to make healthier choices is essential.

## 6.4 Assessing health needs

In order to develop appropriate policies and strategies, we need to understand how to establish what the need is. Bradshaw (1972) identified four types of social need: comparative, felt, expressed and normative. This is a helpful initial tool for exploring what the needs are. *Table 6.1* sets out the meaning of each need and provides an example to illustrate this meaning. We can see that the need may be individual, community or population based.

**Table 6.1** *Four types of social need (adapted from Bradshaw, 1972)*

| Need | Meaning | Example |
|---|---|---|
| Comparative | This need compares similar individuals or groups with others to identify whether they receive the same as each other | Comparing geographical areas where one has a high incidence of lung cancer and the other does not |
| Felt | The individual has a perceived need; a limitation of this is that their perceived need will be limited by their level of knowledge and understanding | A service user (patient/client) has pain in their hip |
| Expressed | This is where the desired need (sometimes a felt need) becomes an action | The wish to give up smoking leads to patient accessing a smoking cessation clinic; or patient visits their GP about the pain in their hip |
| Normative | These are needs that are defined by experts but may differ according to the expert | Immunisations and vaccinations |

*Chapter 6: Building a healthy public policy*

> ### ACTIVITY 6.6
> Think of another example for each need and write them in the table below.

| Need | Example |
|---|---|
| Comparative | |
| Felt | |
| Expressed | |
| Normative | |

Subsequently further definitions and models of health needs have been developed. For example, Cavanagh and Chadwick define health needs assessment (HNA) as:

> … a systematic method for reviewing the health issues facing a population, leading to agreed priorities and resource allocation that will improve health and reduce inequalities.

(Cavanagh and Chadwick, 2005, p. 3)

They identify the benefits of undertaking an HNA as:
- *Strengthening community involvement in decision making*
- *Improved public patient participation*
- *Improved team and partnership working*
- *Professional development of skills and experience*
- *Improved patient care*
- *Improved communication with other agencies and the public*
- *Better use of resources*

(Cavanagh and Chadwick, 2005, p. 7)

The following are examples of differing models for undertaking an HNA (Harvey and Taylor, 2013):
- Epidemiological HNA – uses quantitative data; for example, the incidence of disease or mortality rates, services provided between differing populations and data relating to the effectiveness of interventions
- Comparative HNA – compares one group with another

- Corporative HNA – this approach might use epidemiological HNA and comparative HNA but also includes the perspectives of professionals, patients/clients and the public; for example, joint strategic needs assessment (JSNA) which is discussed later in this chapter.

The following case study provides an example of how an HNA such as the model cited above was used to expand one hospice's provision of care.

### CASE STUDY 6.1 USING HNA TO EXPAND HOSPICE-BASED PALLIATIVE CARE PROVISION

A hospice in London that serves the population of Greenwich and Bexley undertook an HNA to demonstrate the need to expand their palliative care provision for people with life-limiting diseases.

At the time the needs assessment was undertaken, the hospice had a day hospice (day care centre) which had fifteen day cases per day, three days a week and a twelve-bedded inpatient unit which provided palliative care, for those in need, within a population of 430 000. The staff comprised one full-time equivalent palliative care consultant, ten registered nurses, ten healthcare assistants and other services such as counselling and complementary therapies. There was a strong contribution to the daily running of the hospice by volunteers.

Information was obtained from local NHS Public Health Reports, Thames Cancer Registry, the then Office of Population Census and Surveys (now known as the Office for National Statistics) death and registration (diseases) data, hospice records and annual reports. *Epidemiological* information that was gathered included demographic details, the level of deprivation in each borough and the incidence and prevalence of cancer and non-cancer diagnosis within Greenwich and Bexley. These were compared with the prevalence of those diseases in the wider local area of south-east England (*Comparative*). Current specialist palliative care provision was reviewed and patients and relatives, as well as hospice staff and volunteers, were invited to give feedback (*Corporative*).

What was clear from the data gathered was that there was an increasing number of referrals and there was regularly a waiting list of fifteen patients for inpatient admission. This added to pressure on beds within the local acute and community NHS Trusts, thereby adding to their waiting lists. The data also demonstrated that there was limited access to the hospice's specialist palliative care services for those with a non-cancer diagnosis and low uptake by some ethnic groups.

A proposal for expansion was drawn up to increase the number of inpatient beds to nineteen, which met the national accepted number of beds per population at that time. Day hospice places were to increase to 30 cases a day. The plans were agreed by the then local health authority. Increased inpatient and day patients led to increasing the workforce to eighteen healthcare assistants, fifteen registered nurses, one part-time medical officer and one part-time consultant to work with the existing consultant. This improved accessibility for the local population and extended the provision to patients with non-cancer diagnoses which ensured equity. The high incidence of lung cancer led to the development of a nurse specialist post in breathlessness. Educational needs were also identified and addressed, such as cultural awareness. Additional funding was also required which led to the further enhancement and promotion of the hospice with open days and increased fundraising.

Adapted from Knight and Meek (2003).

Since the implementation of the Local Government and Public Involvement in Health Act (HM Government, 2007), localities (defined areas) must produce their own JSNA. This informs the funding and development of suitable and effective local health and social services to meet their local needs. Those involved in undertaking the JSNA include the local authority (including representation from the local public health department), local NHS, service users (patients/clients) and community organisations (for example, non-governmental organisations and charities such as MIND or local hospice). They all work together to assess the local population needs and then plan for future needs to reduce health inequalities and improve the health of their local population (health outcomes).

### ACTIVITY 6.7

Search the internet to find the JSNA for the locality in which you are working and identify what the specific needs are and how these needs will be met. If you live in a different locality, find that JSNA and compare them. What are the differences? Are there similarities?

Cavanagh and Chadwick (2005, p. 21) identify five steps when undertaking an HNA:
- Step 1: **Getting started**. This involves identifying the population, deciding on the aim of the HNA and who needs to be involved, identifying the resources and any risks.
- Step 2: **Identifying health priorities**. This is achieved by describing the chosen population (for example, by age, gender and so on), gathering the relevant data including the perceived needs and then identifying and assessing health conditions and determining factors; for example, access to clinics.
- Step 3: **Assessing a healthy priority for action**. This involves selecting the largest and most severe health conditions and determining factors and specifying the most effective and appropriate interventions and actions needed. For example, see *Case study 6.1*.
- Step 4: **Planning for change**. It is important to clarify aims of the identified intervention, set up an action plan for its implementation and ensure there is ongoing monitoring while the interventions/actions are ongoing, alongside evaluating them. A risk management strategy is also needed.
- Step 5: **Moving on/review**: This involves identification of what has been learnt, what the impact has been (discussed in *Section 6.5*) and then choosing the next health priority.

## 6.5 Health impact assessments

The WHO (2019) defines a health impact assessment (HIA) as *"a means of assessing the health impacts of policies, plans and projects in diverse economic sectors using quantitative, qualitative and participatory techniques"*. What this means in practice is that an HIA provides a way in which to examine what the possible impact would be of a *"policy, programme or project on a population, particularly on vulnerable or disadvantaged groups"* (WHO, 2019).

The intended outcome is to ensure that it not only enhances health, but also that the adverse risk is the lowest possible (WHO, 2019). The findings and recommendations are presented to those making the decision and those who have an interest in them; for example, NHS, local authority and voluntary organisations such as charities and non-governmental organisations (stakeholders).

There are four values that underpin an HIA that the policy, programme or project needs to include: people who it will affect, equity among the identified population, use of the best available evidence from research (quantitative and qualitative) and sustainability (WHO, 2019). An HIA can inform both local and national policy making and projects.

An example is the HIA undertaken for the Greater London Authority, relating to air pollution and asthma in London. This demonstrated that asthma was exacerbated when associated with air pollution and found that children were more at risk than adults (Walton *et al.*, 2019). Children with acute asthma attacks were reported to make up a quarter of all hospital admissions in London. The evidence used as a basis for this HIA identified that the link between air pollution and asthma is associated with nitrogen dioxide, diesel particulate matter and the closeness to traffic (Walton *et al.*, 2019).

### ACTIVITY 6.8

If you were the Mayor of London and responsible for leading policy making, what decisions and policies would you make to reduce the exacerbation of childhood asthma associated with air pollution?

## 6.6 Developing health literacy within populations

A helpful definition of health literacy is that it:

> … *implies the achievement of a level of knowledge, personal skills and confidence to take action to improve personal and community health by changing personal lifestyles and living conditions. Thus, health literacy means more than being able to read pamphlets and make appointments. By improving people's access to health information, and their capacity to use it effectively, health literacy is critical to empowerment.*
>
> (WHO, 1998)

Hence, health literacy is about having the resources and ability to meet challenges and make changes to enhance one's health.

### ACTIVITY 6.9

Re-read the Ottawa Charter's definition of health promotion in *Section 6.1*.

Reflect on this and the definition for health literacy and consider what the term 'empowerment' means to you.

Do you feel empowered to make changes to enhance your own health and wellbeing?

Empowerment of individuals, families and communities is essential for health behaviours to change and to reduce health inequalities. Naidoo and Wills (2016, p. 75) define empowerment as *"the act of acquiring power and the ability to make decisions and take control over one's life"*. For health professionals, this is a challenge. For example, we know the potential impact that smoking can have on an individual's health. However, we can give information (for example, a leaflet (health education)) but we cannot make the individual give up smoking. What we can do is encourage and empower them to make an informed choice which includes providing information that is person-centred with clear signposting to services. In addition, we need to support them to develop their self-esteem (their perception of their value and confidence), their self-efficacy (the belief that they have the ability and resources to act and change their health behaviour) and to understand their locus of control (the belief they have control over their lives – internal locus of control) rather than feeing they are powerless (external locus of control).

> **ACTIVITY 6.10**
>
> Return to *Chapters 2* and *3* and remind yourself of the earlier discussions in this book regarding empowerment in relation to health promotion and health inequalities.

There are many models/tools for promoting the health literacy of the population and some are briefly outlined here.

### 6.6.1 The health belief model

The health belief model initially devised by Rosenstock in 1966, then later modified by Becker in 1974 (Strecher and Rosenstock, 1997), acknowledges that everyone has their own personal beliefs and that these are an important part of their decision-making. In this model, the individual weighs up the pros (advantages) and cons (disadvantages) of taking an action to boost their health. This is an important model; for example, in relation to sexual health, immunisation and vaccination programmes. The decision is based on the individual's appraisal of the following:

- perceived susceptibility (*Am I vulnerable?*)
- perceived severity (*Am I at risk or in danger?*)
- perceived benefits (*What are the advantages for me?*)
- perceived barriers (*What are the disadvantages and what are my obstacles?*)
- cue to action (*What is prompting me to act?*)
- their self-efficacy.

(adapted from Strecher and Rosenstock, 1997, pp. 113–14)

Using the health belief model, we can reflect on how it relates to immunisation and vaccination. For example, measles is a viral disease that can cause neurological (brain) damage and death (PHE, 2013). An immunisation programme is available for MMR, given around the child's first birthday with a second dose at three years four months of age or soon after (PHE, 2013). Young people are also offered the MMR vaccine if they have not had the two doses (PHE, 2013). Separate or single measles vaccinations are also available.

Since 2016, the UK had been considered as a measles-free country owing to the high vaccination rate which provided immunity from the disease for the person who receives it. In addition, those who are vaccinated are less likely to infect those who have not been vaccinated and this provides 'herd immunity' (PHE, 2013). Herd immunity is achieved when 95% of the population have been vaccinated (Ford, 2019).

In 2019, the UK lost its measles-free status as a result of there being 231 confirmed cases of measles in the first three months of 2019 (Ford, 2019) and, therefore, no longer had 'herd immunity' due to the reduced uptake of the vaccination. Not taking up vaccinations may be due to parental choice or for medical reasons. There also remain public concerns, despite evidence to the contrary, regarding a purported link between the MMR vaccine and the child developing autism, even though research suggesting such a link has been thoroughly discredited. For more information see the 2019 NHS article, *'No link between MMR and autism,' major study finds*, available at: bit.ly/6-6-1.

Using the example of measles, we can explore the health belief model in *Table 6.2* in relation to whether a parent/carer would permit their child to have the MMR vaccine.

**Table 6.2** *The health belief model*

| | |
|---|---|
| **Perceived susceptibility** | "I don't know anyone who has had measles"<br><br>"It is only a childhood disease" |
| **Perceived severity** | "Is my child really at risk of getting measles?"<br><br>"There is an outbreak of measles in the area where I live"<br><br>"No one I know has died or has brain damage from measles" |
| **Perceived benefits** | "This will protect my child from being ill with measles"<br><br>"This will protect my friend's child who cannot have the MMR vaccine" |
| **Perceived barriers** | "I have no transport to the immunisation and vaccination clinic"<br><br>"I work full-time and the clinic is not open when I am able to go"<br><br>"I do not want my child to be in pain when they have the injection"<br><br>"Do I have to pay?" |

| | |
|---|---|
| **Cue to action** | There is a local outbreak of measles |
| | The national or local news reports that a child has died as a result of measles |
| | There is a social media campaign about the risk of a child developing measles, and promoting the MMR vaccine |
| | The national government decides to make immunising the child compulsory before they can attend school* |
| **Self-efficacy** | "I can arrange time off work" |
| | "The vaccination is free" |
| | "I can ensure I have some pain relief for my child in the house" |
| | "The bus stops right outside the clinic" |
| | "My friend will give me a lift to the clinic" |

\* In September 2019, a statement was made that the UK government was considering compulsory vaccination and the NHS is considering making the MMR vaccine available to be administered in supermarkets and town centres to increase accessibility.

### 6.6.2 The theory of reasoned action

Similarly to the health belief model, Ajzen and Fishbein's (1980) theory of reasoned action, which was introduced in *Chapter 2*, proposes that an individual's behaviour is influenced by their attitude towards the behaviour. In addition, they acknowledge that social 'norms' play an important role in an individual's decision-making. For example, an individual's attitude may be that they know that giving up smoking is beneficial to their health. However, their perception of what is 'normal' is based on their friendships, family, community, education and culture and whether they want to fit in with these norms, or not, which will influence any action taken.

Consider, if you smoke, it may be that all your friends smoke and you feel that if you give up smoking you will lose this social network as you no longer meet their social 'norms'. Therefore, your attitude and perception of your 'social norms' informs your intent to act (in this case whether to give up smoking or not). If the friendship group all gave up smoking at the same time, then this would influence you to stop smoking as you would wish to fit in with the group's new 'social norms'. Peer pressure, or the influence of a significant person in our lives (e.g. parent, partner or child), is a strong influence on how we will act in order to change our behaviour. This means that it is difficult for a health or social care professional to predict what we, or others, may choose to do.

> **ACTIVITY 6.11**
>
> Think of a health behaviour that you would like to change. What influences can you think of that affect your decision about making this change?

### 6.6.3 The stages of change model

The transtheoretical model is known as the 'stages of change' model. As this title suggests, it describes the process of change in five stages. Embedded in the model is the assumption that change takes time and planning and is not a 'spur of the moment' decision (Prochaska and DiClemente, 1986). The model also identifies that changing health behaviour is not a process that follows a straight line. People may move backwards and forwards through the different stages until they achieve a permanent change in their behaviour. This means that we need to accept that they may relapse into their previous health behaviour. However, this does not mean that they will not eventually achieve their desired change. It also means that we need to consider that, as health and social care professionals, we may need a different approach for each of the five stages.

The five stages are presented in *Table 6.3* with an explanation of each stage, together with an example and an example of a suggested approach that a health professional may adopt in a health promotion context.

**Table 6.3** *The stages of change model*

| Stage | Explanation | Example | Examples of suggested approaches * |
|---|---|---|---|
| Pre-contemplation | The individual does not feel that there are any changes to their lifestyle and health behaviours that they need to make | "My dad smoked 40 cigarettes a day and he lived to 92" | Non-directive communication, empathy, raise awareness of the harm caused by smoking |
| Contemplation | The individual is considering making a change. They may be thinking about the health risks associated with their behaviour but may not be ready to make that change<br><br>They may be asking for information | The individual is aware of the risks of smoking and is thinking about the pros and cons of stopping smoking | Active listening, non-directive and non-judgemental communication to enable them to highlight for themselves the benefits of stopping smoking, empathy, building their self-efficacy and self-esteem<br><br>May need to provide information and signpost to smoking cessation services |

| | | | |
|---|---|---|---|
| Preparing to change | The individual has decided that they are going to make a lifestyle change

They have decided what their goal is but may not know what steps to take | The decision is made to stop smoking

They may ask for advice and guidance or seek this information themselves (e.g. on the internet) or from family and friends | Support the individual to make a plan to stop smoking (e.g. using SMARTER, as discussed later in this chapter), negotiate, provide encouragement |
| Making the change | Here the individual is committed to make the change and undertakes the action to achieve it | Attending a smoking cessation clinic | Encourage reflection on achievements to date, praise, be empathetic and non-judgemental |
| Maintenance | The individual achieves the change and the new behaviour is achieved

Sustained behaviour change is usually considered to be 6 months or more | The individual stops smoking | Praise and support |

*With thanks to Nikki Glendening at Bournemouth University

The model accepts that individuals may relapse and that this is not a failure on their part; for example, an individual decides to stop smoking but is then made redundant after a month and decides to start smoking again. When their life is stable, they may choose to try to stop smoking again and this time they may be successful for longer or it may be a permanent change. A further example of how the stages of change model can be applied in practice is provided in *Chapter 2*.

### ACTIVITY 6.12

Think about a health promotion intervention/activity that you have observed or been involved with in your clinical practice.
- What stage do you think the individual was at?
- Was the health professional's approach appropriate for that stage?
- What could have been done differently?

### 6.6.4 Motivational interviewing

In our role as health professionals, telling people what to do does not result in them changing their health behaviour (HEE, 2017). We need to empower them to make the change. Motivational interviewing can help with this and can be defined as *"a non-directive client-based counselling style"* (Naidoo and Wills, 2016, p. 149) as also seen in *Chapter 2*. An example of this is Making Every Contact Count (MECC) which:

> … *supports the opportunistic delivery of consistent and concise healthy lifestyle information and enables individuals to engage in conversations about their health at scale across organisations and populations.*
>
> (PHE, NHS England and HEE, 2016, p. 6)

As an evidence-based model, MECC is currently being rolled out in England and Wales. It provides a person-centred approach to discussing with people their own health and wellbeing and what is important to them. It is an approach that can be used at every stage of Prochaska and DiClemente's (1986) stages of change model, discussed previously.

It is based on the following four behavioural principles:
- *People are responsible for their own choices.*
- *Being given information alone does not make people change.*
- *People come to us with solutions.*
- *It is not possible to persuade people to change their habits.*

(HEE, 2017, p. 10)

There are two levels of MECC interventions:
- MECC level 1: (very brief intervention)

This lasts between 30 seconds and two minutes and provides enough time for the patient/client to identify a health issue and for the health professional to provide support, encouragement and signpost to relevant resources, e.g. a smoking cessation clinic if the individual has identified they wish to give up smoking (PHE, NHS England and HEE, 2016).

- MECC level 2: (brief intervention)

This is longer than two minutes and can last up to five minutes. PHE, NHS England and HEE (2016, p. 15) explain that this *"involves oral discussion, negotiation or encouragement, with or without written or other support or follow-up. It may also involve a referral for further interventions, directing people to other options, or more intensive support"*.

At the core of a successful MECC encounter is the ability to facilitate effective communication in order to hold a conversation which is based on the person's own health needs and goals. The emphasis is on the individual deciding what is important to them and not the health professional. The use of open questions, especially beginning questions with 'How…?' and 'What…?', is essential so that relevant information can be obtained in order to signpost appropriately, support them and assist the individual to set a goal (HEE, 2017). MECC uses the SMARTER framework (Specific, Measurable, Achievable, Relevant, Time-bound, Evaluation and Reviewed) for goal setting (HEE, 2017).

> **ACTIVITY 6.13**
>
> Think of a health behaviour goal that you would like to change for yourself, e.g. eating your 5-a-day fruit and vegetables. When you have chosen your goal, use the SMARTER model to organise how you intend to achieve this goal (HEE, 2017).
>
> **S**pecific:
>
> **M**easurable:
>
> **A**chievable:
>
> **R**elevant:
>
> **T**ime-bound:
>
> **E**valuation:
>
> **R**eview:

Further details regarding motivational interviewing, MECC and goal setting can be found in *Chapter 2*.

> **KEY LEARNING POINTS**
>
> Four key points to take away from *Chapter 6*:
> - All policies and legislation should aim to maintain and enhance health.
> - Building a public health policy involves all health and social care workers and service users, as well as requiring collaborative and integrated working between the NHS, the public health departments and public health teams, local authorities and the voluntary sector working with local communities.
> - The health needs of a population or community, as well as potential impact, must be identified in order to develop appropriate policies and strategies.
> - There is a range of tools and models that can be used which ensure that person-centred or community-centred approaches can be provided to enhance health literacy and improve health outcomes.

# REFERENCES

Acheson, D. (1988) *Public Health Services*. Available at: www.euro.who.int/en/health-topics/Health-systems/public-health-services (accessed 15 May 2020)

Ajzen, I. and Fishbein, M. (1980) *Understanding Attitudes and Predicting Social Behavior*. Prentice-Hall.

Bradshaw, J. (1972) 'A taxonomy of social need'. In McLachlan, G. (ed.) *Problems and Progress in Medical Care: essays on current research*, 7th series. Oxford University Press, pp. 71–82. (Available at: http://eprints.whiterose.ac.uk/118357/1/bradshaw_taxonomy.pdf (accessed 15 May 2020)

Cavanagh, S. and Chadwick, K. (2005) *Summary: health needs assessment at a glance*. Available at: https://nursingwithacommunityfocus.weebly.com/uploads/6/3/8/1/6381528/health_needs_assessment._a_practical_guide.pdf (accessed 15 May 2020)

Dahlgren, G. and Whitehead, M. (1991) *The Dahlgren–Whitehead Rainbow*. Available at: https://esrc.ukri.org/about-us/50-years-of-esrc/50-achievements/the-dahlgren-whitehead-rainbow/ (accessed 15 May 2020)

Faculty of Public Health (2016) *Good Public Health Practice Framework 2016*. Available at: www.fph.org.uk/media/1304/good-public-health-practice-framework_-2016_final.pdf (accessed 15 May 2020)

Ford, S. (2019) *Loss of 'Measles Free' Status by UK Sparks Widespread Concerns*. Available at: www.nursingtimes.net/news/primary-care/loss-measles-free-status-uk-sparks-widespread-concerns-19-08-2019/ (accessed 15 May 2020)

Harvey, J. and Taylor, V. (2013) *Measuring Health and Wellbeing*. Learning Matters.

Health Education England (2017) *Healthy Conversation Skills: training manual*. HEE.

HM Government (1974) Health and Safety at Work etc. Act 1974. Available at: www.legislation.gov.uk/ukpga/1974/37 (accessed 15 May 2020)

HM Government (2006) Health Act 2006. Available at: www.legislation.gov.uk/ukpga/2006/28/contents (accessed 15 May 2020)

HM Government (2007) Local Government and Public Involvement in Health Act 2007. Available at: www.legislation.gov.uk/ukpga/2007/28/contents (accessed 15 May 2020)

Knight, A. and Meek, F. (2003) Needs assessment: a tool for hospice expansion. *International Journal of Palliative Care*, **9(5):** 195–201.

Naidoo, J. and Wills, J. (2016) *Foundations for Health Promotion*, 4th edition. Elsevier.

Prochaska, J. and DiClemente, C. (1986) 'Toward a comprehensive model of change'. In Miller, W. and Heather, N. (eds) *Treating Addictive Behaviors: processes of change*. Plenum Press.

Public Health England (2013) *The Green Book*. Available at: www.gov.uk/government/collections/immunisation-against-infectious-disease-the-green-book (accessed 15 May 2020)

Public Health England, NHS England and Health Education England (2016) *Making Every Contact Count (MECC): consensus statement*. Available at: www.england.nhs.uk/wp-content/uploads/2016/04/making-every-contact-count.pdf (accessed 15 May 2020)

Strecher, V. and Rosenstock, I. (1997) 'The Health Belief Model'. In: Baum, A., Newman, S., Weinman, J., West, R. and McManus, C. (eds) *Cambridge Handbook of Psychology, Health and Medicine*. Cambridge University Press.

Walton, H., Dajnak, D., Evangelopoulos, D. and Fecht, D. (2019) *Health Impact Assessment of Air Pollution on Asthma in London*. Available at: www.london.gov.uk/sites/default/files/asthma_kings_report_april_2019_final.pdf (accessed 15 May 2020)

World Health Organization (1986) *Ottawa Charter for Health Promotion*. Available at: www.euro.who.int/__data/assets/pdf_file/0004/129532/Ottawa_Charter.pdf?ua=1 (accessed 6 May 2020)

World Health Organization (1988) *Adelaide Recommendations on Healthy Public Policy*. Available at: www.who.int/healthpromotion/conferences/previous/adelaide/en/index1.html (accessed 15 May 2020)

World Health Organization (1998) *Health Literacy*. Available at: www.who.int/healthpromotion/health-literacy/en/ (accessed 15 May 2020)

World Health Organization (2019) *Health Impact Assessment*. Available at: www.who.int/heli/impacts/hiabrief/en/ (accessed 15 May 2020)

# Chapter 7
# Advocating mental health promotion

Gemma Stacey-Emile

> **LEARNING OUTCOMES**
>
> When you have finished this chapter, you should be able to:
>
> **7.1** Define mental health, wellbeing and mental health promotion
>
> **7.2** Discuss issues and barriers that individuals experience which impact on their mental health and wellbeing
>
> **7.3** Identify the importance of individualised mental health promotion and how this can be adapted to encourage personal growth, self-purpose and wellbeing
>
> **7.4** Identify key mental health policies and strategies that can support mental health and wellbeing
>
> **7.5** Outline how you can advocate for good mental health and reduce associated stigma.

## 7.1 Introduction

In the UK, it is believed that one in four adults and one in ten children experience a mental health issue from all walks of life (NHS England, 2020).

The aim of this chapter is to explore definitions of mental health, the meaning of 'mental health and wellbeing' and the impact it has on individuals and the general population. The focus will be on how healthcare professionals advocate *good* mental health and what skills and strategies can be utilised to help achieve this. Barriers and challenges will be explored, along with further examples of how to build and enable others to have an increased sense of positive mental health and wellbeing. It is important that we take every opportunity as healthcare professionals to engage in conversations about mental health to help reduce stigma and raise awareness of services and provision.

## 7.2 Frameworks of perceptions of self and others

Understanding who we are is vital before we can offer advice to others. Benner (2012) reflects on her earlier work for nursing 'from novice to expert' and highlights how expert nurses use their intuition in clinical practice which is based on their practice experience. This knowledge of practice is referred to as 'tacit' or 'intuitive'; through your career you will move from novice to expert, gaining 'conscious and unconscious incompetence and competence'. There is also an expectation that learning will be progressive and lifelong and underpinned by evidence as you continue throughout your career (NMC, 2018).

> **ACTIVITY 7.1**
>
> Think about your training so far. How has your learning changed to date? For example, on your first placement, how did you find giving a handover about a patient to the next shift? How have you developed your communication skills throughout your placements?

At the beginning of your career, while tacit knowledge and intuition are growing and developing, being aware of your capabilities and proficiencies is important for the safety of others. It is also important to recognise personal limitations, seeking help when you are unsure of your practice. For example, the first time you hand over to your colleagues you need to be prepared and offer a logical, clear, concise background so that you do not miss out any key information which could cause harm to the patient.

### 7.2.1 Building self-awareness

Self-awareness and emotional intelligence are key to supporting mental health and wellbeing. As adults there is a sense of assuming that we know who we are and what we want in life using goals, dreams and ambition to drive and motivate us. We can, however, draw on different approaches and evidence to consider why some people appear to find this easier than others, which can assist us when working with patients with specific issues such as depression or psychosis. Oelofsen (2012) identifies the need to explore how practitioners in healthcare absorb the distress of others, including boundaries, and the importance of reflecting on our emotions regularly, as this impacts on how we deliver care to others.

### 7.2.2 Inner and outer self

It is assumed that being 'self-aware' means that we are conscious of our character, how we are perceived by others, and that we are in touch with our beliefs, values, strengths and weaknesses. However, Burnard (1992) emphasises the need to distinguish between one's inner and outer self, incorporating how we feel and what other people see, including our appearance and verbal and non-verbal behaviour.

Developing self-awareness can be complex, but, through clinical supervision and reflecting and learning through practice, having difficult conversations about our behaviour is important for personal growth and development. For example, you may feel you are being assertive and making your point, but to the nursing team/patient you may have come across as bossy and dismissive. This behaviour is fed back through supervision and reflected on in practice. Developing self-awareness also takes courage and confidence. Intrapersonal skills that are needed within mental health nursing and caring for people with mental health issues, need to be acquired through practice, self-development and reflective learning (Howatson-Jones, 2016).

> **ACTIVITY 7.2**
>
> Think about any situations in practice where you have been made aware of something that you did that made you more self-aware of your behaviour and resulted in a change in your practice and/or behaviour.

People with severe and long-term mental health problems may have had a significant amount of contact with healthcare services and some of their contact may not have been positive. Due to the nature of, and stigma associated with mental health it is really important that we consider how we communicate. We should engage with and care for all people with respect, compassion and humanity, but it is important to consider people's vulnerabilities and adjust our behaviour and communication skills accordingly; this is a key nursing skill (Pilgrim, 2020).

### 7.2.3 Johari window

A useful model to consider when working and caring for people is that of the Johari window, developed by psychologists Luft and Ingham (1955), which provides a technique that allows people to understand their relationships with themselves and others. It allows people to identify their strengths, weaknesses and blind spots. The authors also recognise the unconscious mind in their model which has four quadrants:

- Open Space: known to yourself *and* known to others
- Blind Spot: unknown to yourself *and* known to others
- Hidden Area: known to yourself *and* unknown to others
- Unknown Area: unknown to yourself *and* unknown to others

This model is useful within healthcare and nursing as it can be used within appraisals, professional development and clinical supervision, allowing a framework for discussion and reflection on how a situation is viewed, reflected upon and learned from. This model indicates that there are parts of the mind that are private, parts that are social or public, but there is also a part of the self that cannot be seen by oneself or others which is the unconscious (unknown) area of the self. As a professional you need to be mindful of this as a barrier and consider ways to adapt your approach to enable people to accept this.

*Chapter 7: Advocating mental health promotion*

> **ACTIVITY 7.3**
>
> Review the Johari window at: bit.ly/A7-3 (also included in *Chapter 10* as *Figure 10.4*).
>
> Look at the four quadrants and think about what you could put in each quadrant in relation to your understanding of you as a nurse. You will need to ask some of your peers/colleagues to see if there are areas that you are not aware of, i.e. those in the blind spot.

### 7.2.4 Emotional intelligence

Emotional intelligence is the ability to recognise, understand and manage your own emotions while recognising how we can influence other people's emotions and behaviour. According to Goleman (1998) and Akerjordet and Severinsson (2004), emotional intelligence also promotes personal growth and professional competence development. Emotional intelligence concerns sensing what others are feeling and handling relationships effectively, contributing a crucial set of skills for responsive nurse leadership (Goleman, Boyatzis and McKee, 2002; Cummings, Hayduk and Estabrooks, 2005).

The models and definitions discussed above provide a framework to consider perceptions of ourselves and how we are viewed by others. Within the health promotion role of nursing, how we talk to and engage with patients, service users and family members is crucial to ensuring high-quality non-judgemental care. Being self-aware and emotionally intelligent are relative and using reflection and supervision within nursing practice can increase knowledge, self-awareness and emotional intelligence. These core nursing skills will improve health promotion practice to foster health promotion and behaviour change to promote positive health and wellbeing.

## 7.3 Overview of mental health and definitions

The WHO (2018) states that *"health is a state of complete physical, mental and social wellbeing and not merely the absence of disease or infirmity"*. The WHO (1986) Ottawa Charter proposes that *"health promotion is the process of enabling people to increase control over, and to improve, their health"*. In the UK, the Department of Health and Social Care (2019) provides policies to lead the nation's health and social care to help people live more independent, healthier lives for longer. Key components to consider here are the context and what professional responsibilities and skills are required to fulfil these goals.

Two key definitions will be used to explore the meaning of mental health and wellbeing:
- *Mental health is defined as a state of wellbeing in which every individual realizes his or her own potential, can cope with the normal stresses of life, can work productively and fruitfully, and is able to make a contribution to her or his community* (WHO, 2018)
- *Mental wellbeing is a dynamic state in which the individual is able to develop their potential, work productively and creatively, build strong and positive relationships*

*with others and contribute to their community. It is enhanced when an individual is able to fulfil their personal and social goals and achieve a sense of purpose in society* (NICE, 2019).

In the UK everyone has a right to care provision for both their physical and mental health needs. All public health authorities, including NHS organisations, have a duty to respect and promote people's human rights (Equality and Human Rights Commission, 2010). Across the UK there are a range of services and provisions but fundamentally everyone should receive the healthcare that is required to live their optimum life.

Members of the royal family promote the Heads Together charity and celebrities share their own experiences of mental health, dementia in the family or substance misuse problems through the media. Social media also targets young people, offering ways to help develop wellbeing and resilience to the pressures of daily life, with different mobile phone apps focusing on stress relief and sleep.

There has also been increased concern for primary school-aged children. This has been evidenced by the NICE consultations on social, emotional and mental wellbeing in primary and secondary education, school-based interventions, physical and mental health and wellbeing promotion and the Mental Health Foundation Campaign 'Mental health is not extracurricular – make it count'. These demonstrate concern for mental wellbeing of young people (Mental Health Foundation, 2018).

In the nursing and healthcare sector a working definition of mental health is required so that care, treatment and prioritisation can be offered depending on the severity of an individual's presentation of symptoms (Kingdon, Rathod and Asher, 2017). People can present with physical health problems such as poor diet, poor sleep, headaches and physical pain, with an underlying issue of mental health-related problems. It is important to consider the person as a whole and provide a holistic approach to nursing and assessment which includes assessing their physical, biological and psychological health.

Ruddick (2013) discusses how nurses are expected to promote health which includes physical and psychological wellbeing. He proposes that:

> *… nurses work in a variety of services and are in an ideal position to promote patients' sense of empowerment and resilience by helping them to acknowledge their resources, rather than focusing on their disability or illness.*
>
> (Ruddick, 2013, p. 35)

Wand (2011) offers a definition for mental health promotion, suggesting that:

> *… mental health promotion … is concerned with achieving positive mental health and wellbeing in the general population as well as addressing the needs of those at risk from, or experiencing, mental health problems.*
>
> (Wand, 2011, p. 131)

> ### ACTIVITY 7.4
>
> Identify what mental health and mental wellbeing mean to you. You can do this on your own or with peers/friends.
>
> Categorise your answers into thoughts, feelings and behaviours.
>
> Consider which answers are easier to share with people close to you, colleagues and strangers. It is important to note here how some of these thoughts are personal and private and difficult to articulate.

## 7.4 Issues and barriers which impact mental health and wellbeing

As previously indicated, talking about our own mental health can be challenging for a variety of reasons; however, it is important to acknowledge that some people find it easier to talk and disclose their feelings regarding mental health issues than others. Addressing mental health is an issue for the whole population and hopefully, in time, stigma will be reduced (Time to Change, 2020).

The role of a nurse provides a privileged platform, with members of the public trusting nurses and healthcare professionals to provide advice and guidance for both their physical and mental health. Healthcare professionals are in a position to hear and listen to people's stories and experiences. As a result, the health professional is required to offer the most appropriate evidence-based intervention to help the person's situation, so it is vital that nurses feel comfortable talking about any mental health issues to act as a role model for society and the local population.

### 7.4.1 Stigma and mental health

As opposed to other fields of nursing, there is still a stigma around mental health within society as previously outlined; therefore it is crucial that all nurses recognise this.

One area where this can be seen in action is through Time to Change, which is a leading charity that is funded by the Department of Health and Social Care, Comic Relief and the National Lottery Community Fund. It is led by Mind and Rethink Mental Illness to promote mental health equality and reduce the stigma and discrimination that surround people with mental health problems (Time to Change, 2020). Its goal is for the population to openly accept that mental health affects everyone and that we have a responsibility to look after our own mental health and to feel able to express to others when their mental health is deteriorating to ensure measures and interventions can be utilised.

### 7.4.2 Behaviour

People present their mental health symptoms in a range of ways, most of which are conscious explanations and complaints, although some people can present symptoms unconsciously through their behaviour. For example, some people may download a mobile app to help with poor sleep patterns while another person may not, resulting in ongoing poor sleep, leading to poor concentration, irritability and feelings of frustration that they may not link to tiredness. The latter group may be unaware of how they are perceived by other people. More examples of behaviour that may be symptoms of mental ill health include being short-tempered, irritable, uninterested or acting out of character, which family members notice and comment on. Personality and emotions can also be affected by a deterioration of mental health and negative feelings of anxiousness, worry and worthlessness which can build over time (sometimes years); the person may never share these feelings with their loved ones or others due to shame, embarrassment or denial (Time to Change, 2020).

### ACTIVITY 7.5

Take some time out and think about people in your care or family who may be displaying some of these symptoms. Have you recognised them before as symptoms of mental health?

## 7.4.3 Seeking help

A significant number of the population will never seek help for their mental health and wellbeing due to the stigma, but as previously suggested, some may seek self-help resources individually or through different organisations (Mental Health Foundation, 2020a).

Some people will never access mental health services within the NHS but may seek help through charities and third sector organisations that are specific to their needs, such as Alcoholics Anonymous or Cruse, for bereavement care. Others may prefer to seek help via services and organisations that relate directly to their needs so they may feel more in control of sharing their feelings that are specifically related to their trauma or experience. Charity websites such as Alcohol Change UK and Drugwise provide information relating to local and national services and run in parallel with NHS initiatives to help people, including free mobile apps such as 'Days Off' which promote alcohol reduction.

Another proportion of people may end up being ill at work and find it difficult to cope with daily activities and experience absence from work due to symptoms such as anxiety, tiredness, poor concentration and alcohol dependence problems (MIND, 2020). It is important to consider the range of mental health problems that can be experienced; these can vary from day-to-day worries that come and go but have little impact on quality of life, to prolonged bouts of anxiety which can have a significant and detrimental effect on someone's quality of life and that of their families and loved ones.

### ACTIVITY 7.6

Identify services that are available within your local area. This can be a useful resource to pass on to people for specific problems, who were not already aware of the services. Remember not everyone uses the internet so it is useful to know what is available for people locally.

### 7.4.3 Biomedical model of care

Within mental health settings across the UK there is a vast range of primary and secondary care mental health services which are predominantly led by psychiatrists. These often provide a more biomedical model of care which can place the patient in the passive role of the recipient of care (Tyrer, 2013; Hyde, 2019).

### 7.4.4 Labelling

Although definitions have been provided above, it is important in your role as a nurse that terms and terminology are thought through and reflected upon. Terms such as mental health, mental ill health, mental disorder, mental health and wellbeing and psychiatry are important to consider. Different professionals (e.g. medics, occupational therapists, physiotherapists) have historically used and debated the usefulness of such terms for the person experiencing a wide variety of symptoms. Each profession will have their own perspective based on different philosophical beliefs and values which are underpinned by their experience and knowledge of working with other disciplines.

The Mental Health Foundation (2020b) states how *"some diagnoses are controversial and there is much concern in the mental health field that people are too often treated according to or described by their label"*. This can have a profound effect on how some people value their life and place in society. Diagnoses remain the most usual way of dividing and classifying symptoms into groups. Common mental health problems include anxiety and depression. Severe mental illness symptoms include people experiencing an altered perception of reality and/or hallucinations which may affect how they think, feel and behave towards themselves and/or others (Chambers, 2017). Kingdon, Rathod and Asher (2017) and Johnstone (2018) highlight that 'labels' or 'diagnoses' such as 'depression' or 'schizophrenia' given to individuals are unhelpful to the person and can be controversial and misused. For example, anxiety and depression can be severe and long-lasting, which can affect people's ability to live a life that is happy and fulfilling, but these labels are often used inappropriately. It is important to remember the definitions above regarding what mental health and wellbeing are for each individual so that judgements are not made; for example, how one person experiences anxiety may not be the same as another person of the same age and sex who has experienced a similar situation.

> **ACTIVITY 7.7**
>
> Think about different people you care for and/or family/friends from different generations. Think about the label that may be used for them and how individuals may react – either positively or negatively – to this. Then think about how as a nurse you can assist people to seek help and reduce the stigma that they may feel due to their social or cultural backgrounds.

## 7.4.5 Prevalence of mental health problems

There are specific groups of people that need particular thought and consideration due to a higher prevalence of mental health problems (including both common and severe mental illness). Within services prioritisation should be given to people:
- who are black, Asian and from minority ethnic groups
- who are refugees and asylum seekers
- with learning disabilities
- with significant physical health problems
- within the lesbian, gay, bi and trans community
- who experience domestic violence and abuse
- who are homeless
- who misuse drugs, alcohol and/or prescribed and over-the-counter medicine.

(Mental Health Foundation, 2020)

A more useful stance for the purpose of this chapter and in providing care is to approach everyone as unique, offering a person-centred approach. This requires emotional intelligence and a range of communication skills required for that specific interaction. It is also key that a person's demographic characteristics are identified within the assessment process to ensure equality in healthcare. As Carl Rogers (2003) identified, people can maintain their wellbeing by being cared for by someone who offers a non-judgemental positive regard.

### ACTIVITY 7.8

Outline factors that may affect people not accessing help and support for their mental health and wellbeing. Identify services that are available in your locality as a resource that you could signpost people to for help.

## 7.4.6 Nurses' mental health

According to HSE (2019), 'nursing' falls under 'caring' and 'professional roles' under the 'Human health and social work activities'. As such, nurses have a higher rate of work-related stress, depression and anxiety than other occupations. The survey emphasises that females are more likely to experience symptoms of stress, depression and anxiety in the age range of 25–54 years, although male rates were not significantly different to the rest of the population (HSE, 2019). These are important issues that need to be deliberated. As nurses caring for others, we need to know how we can care for ourselves and our peers.

## 7.5 Individualised mental health promotion

Mental health promotion can take many forms, including conversations using the principles of 'Making Every Contact Count (MECC)' (HEE, 2020) discussed in *Chapter 2*. The conversation needs to be non-judgemental, opportunistic and should offer practical advice. It may include signposting to other services and encouragement for people to make positive steps towards a lifestyle change regarding their physical and/or mental health (HEE, 2019). For example, knowing what mental health and wellbeing services and organisations are available locally may help people feel more able to access and seek help, while also encouraging them to take some responsibility for their own health needs.

Life expectancy for people with severe mental illness is reduced by 10–20 years. However, approaches such as MECC, which has a clear positive evidence base for supporting those with common mental health problems (HEE, 2020) are of some use in increasing life expectancy in this group. However, nurse-led interventions and peer support interventions/initiatives show a greater impact for this group, so careful consideration must be given to the individual's needs (Barber and Thornicroft, 2018).

Within holistic assessment the areas below need to be explored. This is important as for some people their stress, anxiety, poor sleep, worry and behaviours are exacerbated because of the impact these have on their day-to-day living. Areas for further consideration during assessments include:
- family
- relationships
- financial problems
- housing
- meaningful activities/work/hobbies.

### 7.5.1 Outcomes Star and Recovery Star

The Outcomes Star and Recovery Star are methods that are widely used within mental health and substance misuse services to collect quality data and information to create a recovery-focused care plan (Mental Health Partnerships, 2019). The 'Star' contains ten areas covering the main aspects of people's lives, including living skills, relationships, work and identity and self-esteem. People set their personal goals within each area and measure, over time, how far they are progressing towards these goals. This can help identify goals and the support required to reach them. Ensuring that progress is achieved, however gradual, can encourage hope. The 4th edition of the Recovery Star (*Figure 7.1*) was revised by Triangle – the original version of the Recovery Star was developed by Triangle in collaboration with the Association of Mental Health Providers, who handed over the role of ensuring hiqh quality use, training, licensing, etc. to Triangle in 2016 (Mental Health Partnerships, 2019).

Both tools record progress in an individual's life domains which include:
- managing mental health
- self-care
- living skills
- social networks
- work
- relationships
- addictive behaviour
- responsibilities
- identity and self-esteem
- trust and hope.

(Mental Health Partnerships, 2019)

## 7.5 Individualised mental health promotion

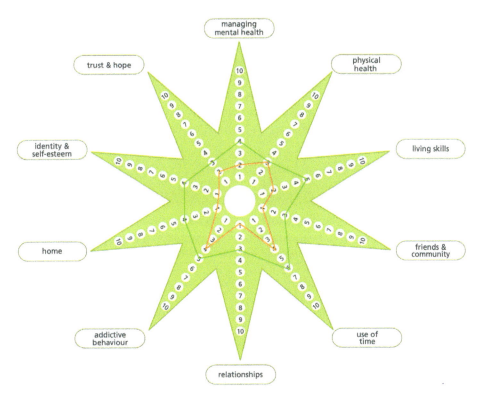

**Figure 7.1** *Fourth edition of the Recovery Star™ © Triangle Consulting Social Enterprise Ltd. Reproduced with permission from Triangle Consulting Social Enterprise Ltd. See www.outcomesstar.org.uk for full copyright details.*

Completing the Star and/or holistic assessment collaboratively is key to promoting ownership of the issues identified. Within nursing, collaboration with patients is crucial and some believe it should be added to the the '6Cs' – care, compassion, courage, communication, competence and commitment (Wiltjer, 2017). Collaboration not only means working with other professionals but also with patients, while respecting each other's autonomy (D'Amour *et al.*, 2008). When there is equal ownership of a stressful aspect of life, devising an individualised approach, goal and plan will enhance the shared decision-making that underpins patient choice.

### 7.5.2 Acceptance and commitment therapy

According to Fledderus (2012), the skills that one learns through acceptance and commitment therapy (ACT) encourage public mental health promotion. If we are emotionally intelligent and self-aware, this reduces the times when thoughts and feelings can overcome us. ACT is an evidence-based philosophical framework that uses acceptance and mindfulness strategies, with commitment and behaviour change strategies, to increase psychological flexibility. ACT is used to provide a positive stance to accept personal feelings, choose a valued course of direction for change and take action on it with regard to setting goals and carrying them out so life can be more meaningful for the person (Hayes, Strosahl and Wilson, 2016).

It is also important when considering ACT services that personal creativity is acknowledged. As Barker, Jensen and Al Battashi (2019) note, mental wellbeing has been linked in many studies to creativity and engagement in creative activities, including in children and young people. Zarobe and Bungay (2017) found that participating in creative activities can have a positive effect on self-confidence, self-esteem, relationship building and a sense of belonging. These qualities have been associated with resilience and mental wellbeing (Zarobe and Bungay, 2017, p. 110).

## 7.6 Policies and strategies that support mental health and wellbeing

There are an array of services and provisions both nationally and globally that support mental health and wellbeing. These include national UK organisations such as Alcohol Change UK and Drugwise and global organisations such as the WHO.

### 7.6.1 UK policies and strategies

The UK government's mental health policy *No Health without Mental Health* provides a strategy for mental health service provision in England (Department of Health, 2011). In Wales, the aims of the 'Together for Mental Health' Delivery Plan 2019–2022 are to focus on improving mental health and wellbeing across all ages with a significant emphasis on the quality and accessibility of mental health services. Another key document by the Welsh Government (2018) is *A Healthier Wales: long term plan for health and social care* which sets out a long-term vision of a 'whole system approach to health and social care', focusing on health and wellbeing and preventing illness. The Welsh Government (2018) identifies the need to further integrate services, promote partnership working and improve holistic approaches to treating physical and mental ill health across the localities.

Scotland has a Mental Health Strategy 2017–2027 which also aims to improve the lives of those living with autism/learning disability, to reduce suicide and to improve access to mental health services for expectant and new mothers. Northern Ireland government services are focusing on mental health and linking this to the Living Well and Healthy Lives Campaign with a joint initiative with the Public Health Agency called *Helping Others* which is a campaign to reach out and support others who may be experiencing mental health problems (Minding Your Head, 2020).

A UK policy report from the Mental Health Foundation (2014), *Mental Health and Prevention: taking local action for better mental health*, provides an overview of what is needed to adopt a 'whole system' approach which includes changing the way society views mental health. It is important to consider current service provision and recognise where there are gaps. There is a need to help local communities to take responsibility, working together to create activities and groups to address local problems experienced by local people. This can be achieved through activities and groups such as cookery groups, promoting healthy eating and physical health, meditation and mindfulness activities instead of offering services for reducing anxiety and weight loss. These community activities can be more inclusive and offered in a more creative way than traditional day services. A move away from self-help groups, for example, to more creative and individual groups such as book clubs, sewing groups or other community groups is being introduced to promote health and wellbeing through a community approach.

> **ACTIVITY 7.9**
>
> Going back to your list of local services in *Activity 7.7* where you identified local organisations, now add to that list any of the above community groups in your area as a resource for patients, carers, family and/or friends.

### 7.6.2 Global action plans

The WHO Mental Health Action Plan 2013–2020 (WHO, 2013) outlined four objectives:
- more effective leadership and governance for mental health
- the provision of comprehensive, integrated mental health and social care services in community-based settings
- implementation of strategies for promotion and prevention
- strengthened information systems, evidence and research.

### 7.6.3 Inequalities in mental illness

*Health Matters: reducing health inequalities in mental illness* (PHE, 2018) outlines the psychosocial pathways that affect us all. The unequal distribution of the social determinants of health includes education, housing and employment. These can further drive inequalities in physical and mental health; the mechanisms by which this happens can be complex and inter-related. Other factors to consider are:
- adverse childhood events, such as being a victim of abuse
- poor housing
- poverty
- traumatic events
- poor working conditions.

Children facing multiple risks have a heightened risk of multiple and sustained childhood mental health difficulties.

Protective factors such as social support and good quality of work and employment conditions can help safeguard against the impact of adverse conditions on poor health (PHE, 2018). According to the Mental Health Foundation (2018), gender, age and differing ethnic groups are key areas to consider. When exploring the barriers that affect people seeking help for their mental health within the community, these factors should be considered. For example, within Wales there are a range of projects underway to make positive differences in raising awareness of additional issues and barriers that face BAME people around accessing mental health services (Diverse Cymru, 2019). This is due to an under-representation of BAME young people accessing mental health services, although statistically this group has a higher incidence of mental health issues than other ethnic groups. The Equality and Human

Rights Commission (2009) outlined some of the specific needs and issues relating to language, religion and culture which may have an impact on how people access mental health organisations, along with other issues that some BAME groups may have experienced, such as stigma and adjustment into western culture.

> **KEY LEARNING POINTS**
>
> Four key points to take away from *Chapter 7*:
> - ✅ Understanding of mental health and wellbeing and mental health promotion is essential in all fields of nursing care.
> - ✅ Awareness of the barriers that individuals experience which impact on mental health and wellbeing, such as stigma and difficulty accessing services, are important to consider when providing health promotion.
> - ✅ Understanding of emotional intelligence, self-awareness and reflection and how these are required in nursing helps provide more individual and person-centred care.
> - ✅ Awareness of the national policies, websites and local facilities/groups can provide useful resources in providing evidence-based up-to-date mental health promotion.

# REFERENCES

Akerjordet, K. and Severinsson, E. (2004) Emotional intelligence in mental health nurses talking about practice. *International Journal of Mental Health Nursing*, **13(3):** 164–70.

Barber, S. and Thornicroft, G. (2018) Reducing the mortality gap in people with severe mental disorders: the role of lifestyle psychosocial interventions. *Frontiers in Psychiatry*, **9:** 463. DOI: 10.3389/fpsyt.2018.00463

Barker, S., Jensen, L. and Al Battashi, H. (2019) *Mental Wellbeing and Psychology: the role of art and history in self discovery and creation*. Routledge.

Benner, P. (2012) Educating nurses: a call for radical transformation – how far have we come? *The Journal of Nursing Education*, **51(4):** 183–4. DOI: 10.3928/01484834-20120402-01.

Burnard, P. (1992) *Know Yourself! Self awareness activities for nurses*. Scutari.

Chambers, M. (ed.) (2017) *Psychiatric and Mental Health Nursing: the craft of caring*, 3rd edition. Routledge.

Cummings, G., Hayduk, L. and Estabrooks, C. (2005) Mitigating the impact of hospital restructuring on nurses: the responsibility of emotionally intelligent leadership. *Nursing Research*, **54(1):** 2–12. DOI: org/10.1097/00006199-200501000-00002

D'Amour, D., Goulet, L., Labadie, J. *et al.* (2008) A model and typology of collaboration between professionals in healthcare organizations. *BMC Health Service Research*, **8:** 188. DOI: 10.1186/1472-6963-8-188.

Department of Health (2011) *No Health without Mental Health*. Available at: https://assets.publishing.service.gov.uk/government/uploads/system/uploads/attachment_data/file/138253/dh_124058.pdf (accessed 18 May 2020)

Department of Health and Social Care (2019) *Corporate report: DHSC single department plan*. Available at: https://www.gov.uk/government/publications/department-of-health-single-departmental-plan/dhsc-single-departmental-plan (accessed 18 May 2020)

Diverse Cymru (2019) *Promoting Equality for All*. Available at www.diversecymru.org.uk/ (accessed 18 May 2020)

Equality and Human Rights Commission (2009) *Human Rights Enquiry 2009*. Available at: www.equalityhumanrights.com/en/our-human-rights-work/human-rights-inquiry-2009 (accessed 18 May 2020)

Equality and Human Rights Commission (2010) Equality Act 2010. Available at: www.equalityhumanrights.com/en/equality-act/equality-act-2010 (accessed 18 May 2020)

Fledderus, M. (2012) *Acceptance and Commitment Therapy for Public Mental Health Promotion*. Universiteit Twente. Available at: https://doi.org/10.3990/1.9789036533133 (accessed 18 May 2020)

Goleman, D. (1998) *Working with Emotional Intelligence*. Bloomsbury.

Goleman, D., Boyatzis, R. and McKee, A. (2002) *Primal Leadership: realizing the power of emotional intelligence*. Harvard Business School Press.

Hayes, S., Strosahl, K. and Wilson, K. (2016) *Acceptance and Commitment Therapy: the process and practice of mindful change*, 2nd edition. Guilford Press.

Health and Safety Executive (2019) *Work-related Stress, Anxiety or Depression Statistics in Great Britain 2019*. Available at: www.hse.gov.uk/statistics/causdis/stress.pdf (accessed 18 May 2020)

Health Education England (2019) *Making Every Contact Count*. Available at: www.makingeverycontactcount.co.uk (accessed 7 July 2020)

Howatson-Jones, L. (2016) *Reflective Practice in Nursing*, 3rd edition. SAGE.

Hyde, J. (2019) 'Understanding and assessing the needs of families and carers'. In Evans, N. (ed.) *Family Work in Mental Health: a skills approach*. MK Publishing.

Johnstone, L. (2018) Psychological formulation as an alternative to psychiatric diagnosis. *Journal of Humanistic Psychology*, **58(1):** 30–46. Available at: https://journals.sagepub.com/doi/10.1177/0022167817722230 (accessed 18 May 2020)

Kingdon, D., Rathod, S. and Asher, C. (2017) 'Classification of mental illness'. In Chambers, M. (ed.) *Psychiatric and Mental Health Nursing*. Routledge.

Luft, J. and Ingham, H. (1955) *The Johari Window: a graphic model for interpersonal relations*. University of California, Western Training Lab.

Mental Health Foundation (2014) *Mental Health and Prevention: taking local action for better mental health*. Available at www.mentalhealth.org.uk/publications/mental-health-and-prevention-taking-local-action-better-mental-health (accessed 18 May 2020)

Mental Health Foundation (2018) *Mental Health in Schools: Make it Count*. Available at www.mentalhealth.org.uk/campaigns/mental-health-schools-make-it-count (accessed 18 May 2020)

Mental Health Foundation (2020a) *Prevention is the Heart of our Work in Mental Health*. Available at www.mentalhealth.org.uk/ (accessed 18 May 2020)

Mental Health Foundation (2020b) *What are Mental Health Problems?* Available at: www.mentalhealth.org.uk/your-mental-health/about-mental-health/what-are-mental-health-problems (accessed 18 May 2020)

Mental Health Partnerships (2019) *Mental Health Partnerships: sharing knowledge, learning and innovation to improve health and care*. Available at https://mentalhealthpartnerships.com/home/about/ (accessed 18 May 2020)

MIND (2020) *Mental Health at Work*. Available at: www.mind.org.uk/workplace/mental-health-at-work/ (accessed 18 May 2020)

Minding Your Head (2020) *Mental Health*. Available at: www.mindingyourhead.info/main-menu/mental-health (accessed 18 May 2020)

National Institute for Health and Care Excellence (2019) *Mental Health and Wellbeing*. Available at: www.nice.org.uk/guidance/lifestyle-and-wellbeing/mental-health-and-wellbeing (accessed 18 May 2020)

NHS England (2020) *Mental Health*. Available at: www.england.nhs.uk/mental-health/ (accessed 18 May 2020)

Nursing and Midwifery Council (2018) *The Code: professional standards of practice and behaviour for nurses, midwives and nursing associates*. Available at: www.nmc.org.uk/standards/code (accessed 6 May 2020)

Oelofsen, N. (2012) *Developing Reflective Practice*. Lantern Publishing.

Pilgrim, D. (2020) *Key Concepts in Mental Health*, 5th edition. SAGE.

Public Health England (2018) *Health Matters: reducing health inequalities in mental illness*. Available at: www.gov.uk/government/publications/health-matters-reducing-health-inequalities-in-mental-illness/health-matters-reducing-health-inequalities-in-mental-illness#inequalities-experienced-by-people-with-mental-illness (accessed 18 May 2020)

Rogers, C. (2003) *Client-Centered Therapy: its current practice, implications and theory*. Constable and Robinson.

Ruddick, F. (2013) Promoting mental health and wellbeing. *Nursing Standard*, **27:** 35–9.

Time to Change (2020) *About us*. Available at www.time-to-change.org.uk/about-us (accessed 18 May 2020)

Tyrer, P. (2013) *Models for Mental Disorder*, 5th edition. Wiley.

Wand, T. (2011) Real mental health promotion requires a reorientation of nursing education, practice and research. *Journal of Psychiatric and Mental Health Nursing*, **8(2):** 131–8. DOI: 10.1111/j.1365-2850.2010.01634

Welsh Government (2018) *A Healthier Wales: long term plan for health and social care.* Available at: https://gov.wales/healthier-wales-long-term-plan-health-and-social-care (accessed 18 May 2020)

Wiltjer, H. (2017) Why collaboration should count as a core value of nursing. *Nursing Times*, **113(12):** 49–50.

World Health Organization (1986) *Ottawa Charter for Health Promotion.* Available at: www.euro.who.int/__data/assets/pdf_file/0004/129532/Ottawa_Charter.pdf?ua=1 (accessed 6 May 2020)

World Health Organization (2013) *Mental health action plan 2013–2020.* Available at: www.who.int/mental_health/publications/action_plan/en/ (accessed 18 May 2020)

World Health Organization (2018) *Mental Health: strengthening our response.* Available at: www.who.int/news-room/fact-sheets/detail/mental-health-strengthening-our-response (accessed 18 May 2020)

Zarobe, L. and Bungay, H. (2017) The role of arts activities in developing resilience and mental wellbeing in children and young people a rapid review of the literature. *Perspectives in Public Health*, **137(6):** 337–47. DOI: 10.1177/1757913917712283

# Chapter 8
# Strengthening community action
Sarah Fry

> **LEARNING OUTCOMES**
>
> When you have finished this chapter, you should be able to:
>
> **8.1** Define the terms community and community action
>
> **8.2** Discuss why it is important to understand community
>
> **8.3** Identify the need for community action
>
> **8.4** Describe approaches to community action
>
> **8.5** Discuss barriers to community action
>
> **8.6** Identify strategies for strengthening community action

## 8.1 Introduction

This chapter will introduce the concept of community and discuss why community is important to health. The idea of a community as central to shaping our views on health will be considered, especially in relation to how an individual may feel when they are part of a community. The community as a place for generating ideas about how to make positive changes to health outcomes will be discussed in the context of community empowerment. By the end of the chapter it will be seen that empowered communities are in a better position to produce sustainable changes for the community, which can improve health outcomes and life chances.

## 8.2 What is a community?

The term community is derived from the Latin word *communis*, meaning 'shared in common' (Moorwood, 2006). Therefore, when we consider what a community is, we can think of it as a group of people who are united in some way or have something shared.

In the modern world this can take many forms. For example, most recently the world of social media has seen new internet communities in the form of Facebook, Twitter and Instagram. Community is also defined by the areas in which we live, work or study, which Neufeld *et al.* (2019) describe as geographical/territorial and relational. People can belong to more than one community; an example of this may be someone who identifies with their geographical location, such as the neighbourhood in which a person lives, and with a relational community, such as a student communicating with their peers using social media. Indeed, in universities students are often encouraged by lecturers to use mobile applications, such as WhatsApp, to support their learning by supporting each other within a student community (Pimmer *et al.*, 2019).

### ACTIVITY 8.1

List which types of communities you belong to.

In this chapter we will be focusing on geographical communities, where action to target health behaviour is often directed.

## 8.3 Why is it important to understand community when discussing health?

Identifying with communities can fulfil a psychological need to feel part of something, which can lead to greater life satisfaction (Neufeld *et al.*, 2019). It is important that this benefit is understood and applied to health improvement strategies. Individuals identify with the normal social behaviour of others in their neighbourhood and this identity can influence a person's health behaviour (Murphy *et al.*, 2018). Therefore, in health-related work, the concept of community is useful for understanding how the way in which people live can affect their health, and how this can be understood across large numbers of people. This applies to rural (Winther, 2017) and urban (Frostick *et al.*, 2017) areas, where the needs of communities can be very different depending on the expectations of the people from the community.

The French philosopher Pierre Bourdieu described the influence of geographical location on behaviour as social capital theory and this can be applied to understanding why some people are disadvantaged in their health outcomes based on where they live (Bourdieu, 1984). Social capital has been described as shaping a person's life chances and Bourdieu theorises that action based in the space (community) in which a person lives can influence that person's social capital and ultimately their health and wellbeing (Grenfell, 2012).

### ACTIVITY 8.2

Think about the community you live in. What is important to people in your community and how might this affect their health?

Social capital theory has been used by researchers in attempts to understand why people in certain communities seem to have worse outcomes compared to others

(Marmot, 2015). To understand how the social space in which people live can affect individual feelings about health, researchers use the term self-rated health to explain how people feel about themselves based on the environment or community around them (Yu *et al.*, 2015; Mohnen *et al.*, 2015; Browne-Yung *et al.*, 2013; Heim, Hunter and Jones, 2011).

Yu *et al.* (2015) asked individuals to rate their own physical and mental health using tools known to be valid for collecting data on self-rated health (GHQ-12 and BHPS (ISER, 2020)). These are questionnaires that ask individuals to indicate on a scale how well they are feeling that day. For instance, the questions would ask a participant to choose a term describing how they feel, which range from very well to very unwell.

### ACTIVITY 8.3

Think back over the last 12 months about how your health has been. Compared to people of your own age, would you say that your health has on the whole been:
- Excellent
- Good
- Fair
- Poor
- Very poor
- Don't know

Yu *et al.* (2015) also measured social capital by asking how often people were in contact with friends, family or people with a shared interest; their community. These researchers found that people were more likely to rate their health highly if they had access to social networks with similar interests and that people who did not have these networks were more likely to have experienced depression. Findings similar to these were described by Browne-Yung *et al.* (2013), who also found that individuals living in a neighbourhood that was socially deprived of community activity or support, rated their health as poor or very poor. This was compared to a neighbourhood that had greater social activity and social links, described as better social capital, who rated their health as good or very good (Browne-Yung *et al.*, 2013).

### ACTIVITY 8.4

Thinking about the work of Yu *et al.* (2015) and their measurement of social capital, how would you describe social capital theory? Write down what you think social capital theory is.

## 8.4 Community action to improve the social environment

We have seen so far that a person's social environment, or their social capital, is important in how they rate their own health, both mentally and physically. We have also discussed that this can be self-rated; it is important to understand how people rate their own social spaces and their health.

It has been suggested that providing communities with the necessary tools to improve their health empowers them to make changes for themselves away from government-led interventions (Capriano, 2008). Examples of these include:
- setting up leisure opportunities for children (Oncescu and Neufeld, 2019)
- setting up gardening groups for local green spaces (Derges *et al.*, 2014)
- creating a community hub for teaching extended skills such as computer technology (Murphy *et al.*, 2018).

This is sometimes referred to as community empowerment and we will come back to this later in the chapter.

An example of a government-led intervention is the smoking ban in the UK. The smoking ban in 2007, part of the Health Act 2006, involved smoking controls in public places, such as work environments, shops and public houses (HM Government, 2006). The approach to implement this meant smoking in such places became illegal, but public engagement with this was at first problematic (Crosby *et al.*, 2018) and the law difficult to implement. Crosby *et al.* (2018) argued that implementation of the smoking ban should have been at a community level, as well as national level (such as police enforcement campaigns), motivating individuals to comply with this new law because they understood the benefits at a community and personal level. Motivating communities to implement the ban may have also led to individuals rating their self-rated health highly, because they were fully engaged with the smoking ban and how this would lead to a healthy environment.

Academics who have taken this individual and community approach to implementing sustainable changes to health include Labonte and Robertson (1996). Labonte and Robertson were among the first academics to consider health promotion and education as a task that should be driven by a community of people. They took the approach that communities should be empowered to make their own decisions about how they can improve their health and their environments and how this can be done with a specific set of social actions. We will now discuss what these social actions might be.

## 8.4.1 Examples of community action

Frostick *et al.* (2017) discussed approaches to improving health by drawing on the ideas of communities of people to decide how they would like to learn about their health. Using this approach with people with a shared interest, such as the area in which they live, can create ideas that are good for their community. Wallerstein and Duran (2006) called this Community-based Participatory Research (CBPR). This method of health research is a way of involving a community in planning interventions that they feel may benefit their neighbourhood the most. Derges *et al.* (2014) used this approach with communities in London by inviting individuals to organise health-related activities as a community. Examples of these activities include:
- training communities to improve their housing with DIY workshops
- providing communities with training on improving their environment by developing and planting community spaces

- identifying local champions as activity-focused trainers to promote physical activity.

More information can be found at bit.ly/8-4-1.

### ACTIVITY 8.5

The hyperlink above gives examples of activities used to increase community engagement with health-related activities. Think about a geographical community you have lived in. This might be where you grew up or where you are living now, if this is different. Using this link, find activities that you think would be used by people in your community. Write down these activities; we will come back to them later.

Derges *et al.* (2014) asked members of the communities involved in these interventions how they felt about the activities and found that communities who were invested in improving their social capital (the environment in which they live) gained the most from the activities they took part in. Derges *et al.* (2014) concluded that a community engagement approach led to better outcomes for the interventions, but that investment in community infrastructure, for example public spaces such as parks, fed into feelings of wellbeing and motivation to engage. Therefore, for Derges *et al.* (2014) community action in improving the spaces in which we live is complex and requires engagement from the community as well as investment in infrastructure.

In Wales, a community-orientated project called Communities First was implemented in 2012 with the aim of delivering community innovation to improve wellbeing in areas of deprivation (Murphy *et al.*, 2018). Murphy *et al.* (2018) studied the benefits of the Communities First programme for the communities involved and found that ideas aimed at improving a community's environment work better when they are generated by the community and developed with staff trained in delivering community projects. An example from this project is an activity to provide a space for communities to come together and discuss ideas, such as placing of a skip for depositing unwanted items in the centre of a local neighbourhood. Using this approach, Murphy *et al.* (2018) found that local residents came together while using the skip and discussed how they could create sustainable activities to improve their social space and ultimately, their social capital.

### ACTIVITY 8.6

Listed below are examples of projects that could help residents come together to discuss what they could do as a community action project. Are any of these similar to the community actions you considered in *Activity 8.5*? Why do you think these activities would work?
- Allow the council access to build new green space in the community.
- Work with the council on planning a use for the green space before work starts.
- Rent out rooms in the community centre for dance classes.
- Talk to the wider community about what classes would be attractive for them in the community centre.

*Chapter 8: Strengthening community action*

- Invite an expert speaker to talk about health problems that may be relevant to the community.
- Set up a central community access point, such as local recycling centre, and encourage people to leave ideas on a graffiti wall about what they think are the main health concerns of the community.
- Invite an expert speaker to talk to the community about the importance of community activity.

## 8.5 Barriers to community action

We have discussed how community action can work to bring people together with the aim of generating opportunities for improving the environment and health. Bourdieu (1984) would say that action to improve a person's environment and health can improve their life chances and their social capital. We have seen from Grenfell (2012) that Bourdieu's social capital theory places the space in which a person lives as central to their health and wellbeing, although sometimes actions to improve this space can be difficult.

As we saw in *Chapter 3*, Sir Michael Marmot, a professor of epidemiology and public health, has written extensively about health inequalities and the worrying statistics relating to mortality and lifestyle related to geographical location. In his book *The Health Gap* (Marmot, 2015), Marmot explains a situation in which he talked to a community group in Liverpool about what they thought of the inequalities they faced and how they might work together to tackle these. The community members considered the summary he had given them about how their neighbourhood might affect their health and how he thought they might be able to help themselves. An example of their responses are as follows:

- *We do not want an outside expert telling us what to do. Our values should determine our goals.*
- *The journey is important as well as the destination. How we get there is important, as is where we want to get.*
- *… we do not want an expert telling us what to measure. Our value driven goals should determine how we measure our success.*

(Marmot, 2015, p. 236)

Marmot (2015) considers this as a learning experience in his approach to helping develop community action. Here, he is explaining a situation in which the community understands that they need to take control of their own activities to improve their environment and ultimately their opportunities and health. However, the communities may lack the resources, in experience, time and money, to implement changes that experts can help with; these are the very experts some communities don't want to engage with to try to effect sustainable changes. So here we have a problem, a barrier to implementing community action that may need time and education to resolve.

## ACTIVITY 8.7

Think about the community and community actions you considered in *Activities 8.5* and *8.6*. Write how you think individuals in your community would respond to your suggestions for community action. What barriers might there be?

Browne-Yung *et al.* (2013) considered that people living in areas that are socially disadvantaged may count themselves as well bonded to their community but have fewer resources to work as a community to improve health outcomes. Browne-Yung *et al.* (2013) comment that people in these communities view themselves as 'getting by' and therefore don't see the need to take action. Of course, this is a perfectly acceptable way to view the space in which one lives and we have seen from Yu *et al.* (2015) that neighbourhood friendships can improve a person's feeling of wellbeing. However, we have also seen in the Marmot Review of health inequalities in England (Marmot, 2020) that women living in an area of social deprivation, will, on average, die 6.1 years earlier than those living in areas of least deprivation, and for men the difference in life expectancy is 7.7 years. Those living in areas of deprivation could have an additional 17 years living with a disability. These years of living with a disability related to poor health, such as obesity-related reduced mobility, may be fewer if community-derived actions are taken to improve people's health and wellbeing. It is, therefore, important to continue to strengthen community action.

Liberato *et al.* (2011) believe community action is further hindered by a top-down approach applied to empowering communities to develop community action. This top-down approach often involves external agencies applying expert opinions on what needs to change and how this change should be applied (Liberato *et al.*, 2011). This can, in turn, lead to apathy from the community, with minimal tangible benefits. This is rather like the experience of Marmot, who found the community wanted to take responsibility for their own health-related actions for the benefit of their own communities. This approach is often referred to as community empowerment and we will discuss this in *Section 8.8*.

A fundamental barrier to developing community action is the short-term availability of experts supporting community efforts to evolve as a place of safety, health and prosperity. This was the experience of Murphy *et al.* (2018) when they reviewed the effectiveness of the Communities First programme in Wales. You will remember that the Communities First programme was developed in 2012 with the aim of delivering community innovation to improve wellbeing in areas of deprivation. We discussed above that this approach seemed to work well in providing opportunities to bring people within a community together to discuss how their community might change. However, Murphy *et al.* concede that there are a "minefield of statutory obligations" (Murphy *et al.*, 2018, p. 31) that need to be tackled before sustainable changes can be made. Examples of these are short-term policy-driven projects that can be weak in their sustainability, especially when community support from project teams comes to an end (Winther *et al.*, 2017).

*Chapter 8: Strengthening community action*

We now need to consider how community action can be strengthened by using approaches that produce sustainable changes for communities wanting to live in an environment that encourages good health and strengthens social capital.

## 8.6 How to strengthen community action

Community empowerment is defined as providing communities with resources to make changes that benefit health and lifestyle (Winther *et al.*, 2017). An example of this is educating individuals within a community about the risks of certain health behaviours, which could lead to health-related messages being generated from within the community and therefore create sustainable changes to health behaviour (Oesterle *et al.*, 2018). Oesterle *et al.* (2018) studied the effects of an approach in seven states of the USA, called Communities That Care (CTC). This is an implementation system that educates individuals to make changes with communities using community approaches, such as actions based on the social norms and expectations of the community. An example of this is The Community Youth Development Study (Fagan *et al.*, 2009), which used the CTC approach to reduce adolescent drug use and antisocial behaviour. This work focused on engaging with community partners over six training workshops during which they were educated on the following:

- assessing community readiness to work with experts
- forming a group of people from the local community who are representative of the diversity in the community
- providing the group with information on local health outcomes to inform the group of the need for community action
- experts to work with the community groups to study evidence-based community actions to aid understanding of why these new actions may be beneficial
- experts to work with the community to implement the community action with commitment and in a manner similar to the evidence base.

(Fagan *et al.*, 2009)

This work means educating community members about the need for community action and the aims of the CTC programme interventions. This requires careful selection of individuals capable of and interested in meeting the objectives laid out by the Community Youth Development Study. These people are often called key stakeholders; we will discuss how these people are identified later in the chapter.

The success of the work by Fagan *et al.* (2009) was measured by the engagement of individuals from the community and the completions of each of the points identified above, as well as participation from the community in the approach to focused programmes to reduce adolescent drug use and antisocial behaviour. The implementation of this programme was successful during the initial phase, when the community seemed most motivated (Fagan *et al.*, 2009). The most successful programmes were implemented in schools and particularly with adolescents at greater risk of adopting poor lifestyle choices, such as drug use. Fagan *et al.* (2009) may have seen some of this success because they targeted a smaller community formed from the wider community; for example, the local school, where it is easier to capture those most in need of community action, in a situation where they are ready to learn and accept health-related messages. This is especially true if these messages are delivered by someone who is known to the community and respected for their knowledge of the community.

In *Activity 8.7* we thought about what the barriers to community action might be. Often people can reduce these barriers to action by engaging with the community. These people are often known as key stakeholders and live within the community, so have a greater understanding of community views and needs. Key stakeholders are interested in helping the community, often because they can see there is a need for change in the community and are well respected by the community because of their status and experience (Fry, 2017). In research aimed at finding out what men in an ethnic minority community knew about prostate cancer and how they would work as a community to understand their risks for this cancer, Fry (2017) accessed three key stakeholders to take part in gaining access to their community. These men were respected by the community for their experience in previous health-related work and their knowledge of how the community lived and the difficulties they might face. The men were also identified as key stakeholders because they were ready to be educated about prostate cancer and pass this information on to men in their community (Fry, 2017).

This approach was also used by Kessing *et al.* (2013) in their study of migrant health behaviour. Migrants can be seen as a community with their specific beliefs about how their community may value and contextualise their health needs (Kessing *et al.*, 2013).

### ACTIVITY 8.8

Outline why you think it is important for nurses to know about how migrant communities think about their health. Next, think about a nurse going into a patient's home to change a dressing on a leg wound. How would the nurse use their knowledge of the patient's migrant community to find out who can help the patient at home until their next visit?

## 8.6.1 What have we learnt so far?

We have learnt that to strengthen community action members of the local community need to be involved in implementing actions to improve the wellbeing of their community and to believe that this needs to be done. Community members want to be educated about the need for change by learning about public health concerns relating to their community. Sometimes people in these communities lack the resources to implement changes and this may be because of a lack of knowledge about the effects of community health behaviour and how action can be taken to improve this. We also know that people want to work together to make changes. This can be seen in the experience of Marmot (2015) and in the implementation of the Community Youth Development Study (Fagan, 2009).

We have also learnt that to engage the community and strengthen community action, key stakeholders need to be involved in implementing change. Key stakeholders need to be ready and motivated to work with the community and to learn from experts about what challenges the communities may face. These challenges also need to be viewed as concerns by the key stakeholders, based on their community experience, so that community actions may be effective and sustainable.

Now consider *Case study 8.1*.

### CASE STUDY 8.1 BACKSTREET

Backstreet is a small community of people based on the edges of a large city. The area has been described as an area of deprivation. Most people who live in Backstreet are on the minimum wage or don't work. The houses are small and packed in tightly together. Most houses are in terraces of eight and are back-to-back with another row of houses. The houses have gardens to the front and these are small and face onto the street. The houses facing the main road have gardens that face onto this road and there is a constant flow of traffic from the main city to the suburbs, including buses, as well as people passing through on foot to get in and out of the city.

The environment is noisy. The average house in Backstreet has five or six people living in a small house with two bedrooms, one toilet and two rooms downstairs, including the kitchen. This lack of space often causes disagreements in the houses, as individuals try to live together in cramped conditions. Most houses have two or three generations living together and this includes young children and teenagers, who need different activities to prevent boredom and unhappiness.

Because the environment at home can be difficult, children and teenagers often go out and meet their friends on the streets. There are a few public areas in Backstreet. There is a green area with a playground and a community centre. Unfortunately, the location of Backstreet means that it is easy for people who don't live there to find the green area and use this as a place to 'hang out'. Some of these people use this space to drink alcohol in the evenings and some take drugs. The accessibility of this activity to the local community means some of the teenagers have started to drink and take drugs. To keep up their supply of drugs, some of the teenagers, and also young adults, have asked the local children to buy drugs from someone outside the community in return for money. This has led to the local children getting into trouble with the police and has also made the area more dangerous because more teenagers have started to carry knives.

A group of adults in the community are angry about what is happening in their community, and especially to their children. The local council and police have used the community centre to provide education about the risks of taking drugs and carrying knives, but it is difficult to engage the community and not many people attend these sessions. The community are suspicious of the police after they have increased the stop-and-search strategy with young men in the area. These men feel they are being victimised. The community is also tired of the local council education sessions because nothing seems to change and the sessions are long and not interactive.

## ACTIVITY 8.9

Address the following questions about this community:
- What are the main concerns the community in Backstreet may face?
- Who in the community is most at risk of problems because of these concerns?
- Why might actions from the local council and the police not be engaging the community?
- Based on what you have read in this chapter, what could you do to help the community make their environment a better place to live?
- How might you engage the community in taking action themselves to make changes to their community?
- Which type of person might be able to motivate the community to take part in action designed to strengthen the community response to making improvements?
- Which type of environment would be most appropriate to deliver this community action?

Consider the following points, which may have developed from your thinking about Backstreet. In Backstreet the community may be at risk of illegal activity relating to drug and knife crime and this could be exacerbated by the lack of space in housing which drives young people away from their families and onto the streets. In Backstreet, these young people have been exposed to drugs and alcohol and the increased police presence could mean the police are seen as interfering with activities that get the young people out of overcrowded housing. To make changes for this local community, activities would need to engage the community, so that they can see the benefits. To do this, an expert would need to work with the community to discuss their views on the problems they may be facing and guide a community-led group in making the changes to reduce the risks to young people.

Nurses are in a good position to help communities in these situations. They are often the first point of contact for health-related concerns in a community, as regular visitors to some people's houses. In Backstreet, this may include mental health, child and adult registered nurses who will have a good understanding of the community issues that may affect a person's health.

> **KEY LEARNING POINTS**
>
> Five key points to take away from *Chapter 8*:
> - Social capital, or the environment in which a person lives, can be enriched by asking the community to develop their own actions based on the social norms of their community.
> - Key stakeholders are often required to carry out community activities because they have an understanding of the challenges their community faces. Nurses are in a good position to find a key stakeholder because they have a good knowledge of the community.
> - Projects led from outside the community may be short-term and not sustainable; including a key stakeholder can improve the sustainability and chances of success of community action.
> - Community members want to be educated about the risks they face in their community and how they can develop programmes to make changes to their environment. Nurses have a good level of knowledge about the risks communities face and are in an ideal position to provide communities with this education, because they may be known to the community.
> - Research continues to be carried out using community engagement strategies and collecting data on how community members feel about their own health and the environment, using self-rating tools.

# REFERENCES

Bourdieu, P. (1984) *Distinction: social critique of the judgement of taste*. Routledge Classics.

Browne-Yung, K., Ziersc, A. and Baum, F. (2013) 'Faking 'til you make it': social-capital accumulation of individuals on low incomes living in contrasting socio-economic neighbourhoods and its implications for health and wellbeing. *Social Science & Medicine*, **85:** 9–17. DOI: 10.1016/j.socscimed.2013.02.026

Capriano, R. (2008) Actual or potential neighbourhood resources and access to them: testing hypotheses of social capital for the health of female caregivers. *Social Science and Medicine*, **64:** 4. DOI:10.1016/j.socsimed.2008.04.017

Crosby, S., Bell, D., Savva, G., Edlin, B. and Bewick, B. (2018) The impact of a social norms approach on reducing levels of misperceptions around smokefree hospital entrances amongst patients, staff, and visitors of an NHS hospital: a repeated cross-sectional survey study. *BMC Public Health*, **18:** 1365. DOI:10.1186/s12889-018-6231. Available at: https://bmcpublichealth.biomedcentral.com/articles/10.1186/s12889-018-6231-x (accessed 18 May 2020)

Derges, J., Clow, A., Lynch, R. *et al.* (2014) 'Well London' and the benefits of participation: results of a qualitative study nested in a cluster randomised trial. *BMJ Open*, **4:** e003596. DOI:10.1136/bmjopen-2013- 003596

Fagan, A., Hanson, K., Hawkins, J. and Arthur, M. (2009) Translational research in action: implementation of the Communities That Care prevention system in 12 communities. *Journal of Community Psychology*, **37(7):** 809–29.

Frostick, C., Watts, P., Netuveli, G., Renton, A. and Moore, D. (2017) Well London: results of a community engagement approach to improving health among adolescent from areas of deprivation in London. *Journal of Community Practice*, **25(2):** 235–52. DOI: 10.1080/10705422.2017.1309611

Fry, S. (2017) Perceptions of prostate cancer risk in White Working Class, African Caribbean and Somali men living in South East Wales: a constructivist grounded theory. PhD Thesis, Cardiff University.

Grenfell, M. (2012) *Pierre Bourdieu: key concepts*, 2nd edition. Routledge.

Heim, D., Hunter, S. and Jones, R. (2011) Perceived discrimination, identification, social capital, and wellbeing: relationships with physical health and psychological distress in a UK minority ethnic community sample. *Journal of Cross-Cultural Psychology*, **42(7):** 1145–64. DOI: 10.1177%2F0022022110383310

HM Government (2006) Health Act 2006: *Part 1, Chapter 1, Smoke-free premises*. Available at: www.legislation.gov.uk/ukpga/2006/28/section/2 (accessed 18 May 2020)

Institute for Social and Economic Research (2020) *BHPS Questionnaire and Survey Documents – Wave 18*. Available at: www.iser.essex.ac.uk/bhps/documentation/pdf_versions/survey_docs/wave18/index.html (accessed 18 May 2020)

Kessing, L., Norredam, M., Kvernrod, A-B., Mygind, A. and Kristiansen, M. (2013) Contextualising migrants' health behaviour – a qualitative study of transnational ties and their implications for participation in mammography screening. *BMC Public Health*, **13:** 431. DOI: 10.1186/147102458-13-431

Labonte, R. and Robertson, A. (1996) Delivering the goods, showing our stuff: the case for a constructivist paradigm for health promotion research and practice. *Health Education Quarterly*, **23(4):** 431–47. DOI:10.1177/109019819602300404

Liberato, S., Brimblecombe, J., Ritchie, J., Ferguson, M. and Coveney, J. (2011) Measuring capacity building in communities: a review of the literature. *BMC Public Health*, **11:** 850. DOI: 1471-2458/11/850

Marmot, M. (2015) *The Health Gap: the challenge of an unequal world*. Bloomsbury.

Marmot, M. (2020) *Health Equity in England: the Marmot review 10 years on*. Institute of Health Equity. Available at: www.health.org.uk/sites/default/files/upload/publications/2020/Health%20Equity%20in%20England_The%20Marmot%20Review%2010%20Years%20On_full%20report.pdf (accessed 6 May 2020)

Mohnen, S., Völker, B., Flap, H., Subramanian, S. and Groenewegen, P. (2015) The influence of social capital on individual health: is it the neighbourhood or the network? *Social Indicators Research*, **121:** 195–214.

Moorwood, J. (2006) *Oxford Latin Desk Dictionary*. Oxford University Press.

Murphy, L., Pickernell, D., Brychan, T. and Fuller, T. (2018) Innovation, social capital and regional policy: the case of the Communities First programme in Wales. *Regional Studies, Regional Science*, **5(1):** 21–39. DOI: 10.1080/21681376.2017.1405740

Neufeld, K., Gaucher, D., Starzyk, K. and Boese, G. (2019) How feeling connected to one's own community can increase support for addressing injustice impacting outgroup communities. *Group Process & Intergroup Relations*, **22(4):** 530–43. DOI: 10.1177/1368430217749881

Oesterle, S., Kuklinski, M., Hawkins, J. *et al.* (2018) Long-term effects of the Communities That Care trial on substance use, antisocial behaviour and violence through age 21 years. *American Journal of Public Health*, **108(5):** 659–65. DOI: 10.2105/AJPH.2018.304320

Oncescu, J. and Neufeld, C. (2019) Low-income families and the positive outcomes associated with participation in a community-based education program. *Annals of Leisure Research*, **22(5):** 661–78. DOI: 10.1080/11745398.2019.1624586

Pimmer, C., Bruhlmann, F., Odetola, T. *et al.* (2019) Facilitating professional mobile learning communities with instant messaging. *Computers & Education*, **128:** 102–12. DOI: org/10.1016/j.compedu.2018.09.005

Wallerstein, N. and Duran, B. (2006) Using community-based participatory research to address health disparities. *Health Promotion Practice*, **7(3):** 312–23. DOI: 10.1177/1524839906289376

Winther, A. (2017) Community sustainability: a holistic approach to measuring the sustainability of rural communities in Scotland. *International Journal of Sustainable Development & World Ecology*, **24(4):** 338–51. DOI: 10.1080/13504509.2016.1224987

Yu, G., Sessions, J., Fu, Y. and Wall, M. (2015) A multilevel cross-lagged structural equation analysis for reciprocal relationship between social capital and health. *Social Science & Medicine*, **142:** 1–8. DOI: 10.1016/j.socscimed.2015.08.004.

# Chapter 9
# Professional responsibilities of the nurse as a health promoter

Nita Muir

> **LEARNING OUTCOMES**
>
> When you have finished this chapter, you should be able to:
>
> **9.1** Outline the Nursing and Midwifery Council's professional requirements for health promotion
>
> **9.2** Demonstrate understanding of the key principles of ethics which relate to health promotion
>
> **9.3** Discuss the role of the nurse as a health promotion role model
>
> **9.4** Identify the political dimensions of health promotion

## 9.1 Introduction

Nurses use a range of knowledge and proficiencies when delivering health promotion. This requires an understanding of health and its determinants, of education and learning theory and finally the ethical and wider political aspects of health. This knowledge is practised by nurses through communication, developing relationships, assessment and political awareness and is underpinned by a values-based stance (Kemppainen, Tossavainen and Turunen, 2013). It is recognised by the Nursing and Midwifery Council (NMC, 2018a, 2018b) that both registered nurses and nursing associates can support people at all stages of their life in their health-promoting decisions and be involved with people at different levels and with different foci. So, for example, a nursing associate may work at an individual level with a person which is at a micro level. A registered nurse, in addition to working at a micro level, may be more involved with working with a community; this is described as the meso level. Registered nurses may also work at the global or policy development level, which is described as the macro level.

> ### ACTIVITY 9.1
>
> To appreciate the broad nature of your health-promoting activity, reflect on your most recent clinical practice and identify how and where you think your health-promoting activity has occurred.
>
> Examples may include:
> - with a patient or client when explaining how they may need to adapt their lifestyle following a change of medication
> - giving a flu vaccination
> - being involved in developing a local gardening community initiative to grow vegetables.

In addition to undertaking an outward health-promoting activity, there is a perceived expectation by the public that your health behaviours influence others in being a role model for the public. This perception is reinforced by the individual professionalism expected by the NMC (NMC, 2018c).

This chapter will address four key dimensions of the professional responsibilities of both the registered nurse (RN) and the nursing associate as a health promoter, which are:
- prioritising people
- practising effectively
- preserving safety
- promoting professionalism and trust

(NMC, 2018d)

You will have explored the associated theory of health promotion throughout this book and this chapter will explore the values base underpinning your health-promoting actions and begin to illuminate the political dimension of health-promoting activities which affect your future practice. However, the first point to consider will be the expectations of you by our professional body.

## 9.2 NMC educational standards

The Nursing and Midwifery Council has developed its expectations of the registered nurse in its *Future Nurse* registered nurse standards (NMC, 2018a). There are twelve explicit proficiencies within platform 2 (Promoting health and preventing ill health) and other health-promoting proficiencies scattered throughout the remaining platforms. Within these standards the nursing student develops health-promoting knowledge and proficiencies expected of the registered nurse. Furthermore, the NMC has affirmed that the nursing associate also has professional expectations, with an identified nine proficiencies in the nursing associate standards (NMC, 2018b).

*Table 9.1* provides an example of how these proficiencies may align with the biomedical, behavioural and socio-environmental view of health that you have already explored in the first two chapters of the book (adapted from Sykes, 2014,

## 9.2 NMC educational standards

p. 45). These approaches are identified as underpinning certain health-promoting activities:

**Table 9.1** *Aligning examples of proficiencies with three approaches to health-promoting activity*

|  | Aim of intervention | Registered nurse proficiency examples | Nursing associate proficiency examples |
| --- | --- | --- | --- |
| Biomedical view of health – absence of diseases | Prevention of ill health, targets the whole population, e.g. screening and immunisation | 2.5 Promote and improve mental, physical, behavioural and other health-related outcomes by understanding and explaining the principles, practice and evidence base for health screening programmes | 2.8 Promote health and prevent ill health by understanding the evidence base for immunisation, vaccination and herd immunity |
| Behavioural view of health – related to lifestyle choice | Focuses on changing individual behaviour and encouraging healthy living, e.g. smoking cessation | 2.4 Identify and use all appropriate opportunities, making reasonable adjustments when required, to discuss the impact of smoking, substance and alcohol use, sexual behaviours, diet and exercise on mental, physical and behavioural health and wellbeing, in the context of people's individual circumstances<br><br>2.10 Provide information in accessible ways to help people understand and make decisions about their health, life choices, illness and care | 2.2 Promote preventive health behaviours and provide information to support people to make informed choices to improve their mental, physical, behavioural health and wellbeing |

| Socio-environmental view – health as a by-product of social, economic and environmental determinants | Aim to create supportive environment for health through influencing local health policy and legislation through lobbying and advocacy activities | 2.2 Demonstrate knowledge of epidemiology, demography, genomics and the wider determinants of health, illness and wellbeing and apply this to an understanding of global patterns of health and wellbeing outcomes | 2.4 Understand the factors that may lead to inequalities in health outcomes |
|---|---|---|---|

### ACTIVITY 9.2

To understand the context of the NMC proficiencies for your own practice, identify the remaining proficiencies for your field of practice and align these with the health promotion approaches that you have already explored. An example may be: as a student nurse on a RN programme, proficiency 2.2 is associated with the socio-environmental view of health.

Then, answer this question: Which is the most common approach referred to within the relevant expected proficiencies?

This activity will have helped you identify the broad range of theoretical approaches you are expected to engage with, both within your nursing course and at registration. In addition to the specific health promotion platform within the education standards, there are other proficiencies across the educational standards for both the RN and the nursing associate which are relevant to health promotion activities such as developing political awareness in platform 5 for the RN and Improving Safety in platform 6 (RN) and platform 5 (nursing associate).

## 9.2.1 Preserving safety and safeguarding

The breadth of expected health promotion activity in the RN and nursing associate roles is reinforced by the NMC *Code of Conduct* (NMC, 2018d). The *Code* directly identifies that all nurses are accountable for engaging in the protection of others and preserving safety for both children and vulnerable adults. Safeguarding adults is about reducing or, ideally, preventing the risk of significant harm from abuse and exploitation and simultaneously supporting people to take control of their own lives by making informed choices (RCN, 2018). There is a clear professional expectation that the nurse has a responsibility to observe, identify, report and record concerns (RCN, 2018).

This approach applies to both vulnerable adults and children in the nurse's care. When dealing with safeguarding of children in child protection the following expectations also occur; these are outlined in the latest governmental policy titled

*Working Together to Safeguard Children* (HM Government, 2018). This policy places the child at the centre of any child protection activity and emphasises that agencies, including nurses, will work together for a positive outcome; it has the following expectations:
- protecting children from maltreatment
- preventing impairment of children's health or development
- ensuring that children grow up in circumstances consistent with the provision of safe and effective care
- taking action to enable all children to have the best outcomes.

Preserving safety and safeguarding are integral to nursing practice and utilise your health-promoting knowledge in identifying what is healthy for an individual client/patient, community or family. This, in turn, will also assist in your ability to identify, report and record concerns. *Case study 9.1* and *Activity 9.3* will explore an example of a category of abuse. This activity will enable you to link these categories to your health promotion knowledge and assist you in determining how you may identify the relevant category. If you need to refresh this knowledge, then access your National Skills Agency account for a review of Safeguarding or the RCN guidance at bit.ly/9-2-1.

### CASE STUDY 9.1  REFLECTING ON A CATEGORY OF ABUSE

You are on placement in a community setting, a minor injury unit, when a young girl enters with her mother with a minor injury. The girl is clearly overweight and finding movement difficult because of this.

### ACTIVITY 9.3

To appreciate how the proficiencies associated with health promotion can enable you to meet the professional requirements of being an RN/nursing associate, explore *Case study 9.1* and consider what the underlying issues may be. Working with your practice supervisor, how would you approach this situation? Might you be interested in exploring whether there is any indication of neglect? What actions would you take and what health-promoting intervention would you deliver?

## 9.3 Ethical issues in health promotion

The previous section began to explore some of the ethics associated with health promotion. Ethics generally leads us to ask questions about how we or others should live our/their lives; what we think is acceptable and what is not. To answer these difficult questions relies on our individual moral beliefs in judging what good or bad behaviour is. In turn, this is influenced by our reasoning, the law, our professional codes and religious beliefs. Essentially through ethics we decide what is right and wrong (Seedhouse, 2004). It is, therefore, important that we understand how ethics work.

## 9.3.1 Ethical frameworks

Authors suggest that ethical frameworks are useful in health promotion as they can guide decision-making. This is particularly important when there is minimal evidence or theoretical context to support interventions (Seedhouse, 2004; Tannahill, 2008). A framework offers a level of consistency between decisions. In the UK, the most common frameworks are based on the four levels of biomedical ethics developed by Beauchamp and Childress (2013):

- At the first level, *Moral judgements* are made in individual cases. In health promotion this relates to how we make decisions about individual behaviour and whether or not this is deemed to be healthy/good behaviour. Moral judgements are based on our own values and beliefs.
- At the second level, *Rules* which state what ought and ought not to be done, are used to justify moral judgements. Beauchamp and Childress (2013) identify that this level is based on being truthful and loyal and respecting a person's privacy and confidentiality. In the context of nursing the Nursing and Midwifery Council has produced the *Code of Conduct* (NMC, 2018d) to frame ethical rules for nurses to abide by.
- Third level *Principles* are the basis for these rules, with principles of: independence (autonomy), being fair (justice), to do good (beneficence) or, at the very least, to do no harm (non-maleficence).
- At the fourth level, *Theories* group the Rules and Principles together under specific theories.

These ethical rules and principles can be applied with differing levels of priority depending on the nature of the scenario.

## 9.3.2 Nursing and Midwifery Council – *Code of Conduct* (2018)

Being a nurse means that we frequently make ethical decisions, although we may not always perceive this. Thinking ethically in the context of nursing and health promotion means we must always put the care of others as our primary concern; this way of thinking and reasoning is guided by our professional rules, code of conduct and the law. To aid in decision-making the code of conduct provides an ethical framework to guide our decision-making and actions when working with areas of activity that may be contentious or problematic (Thomson, 2010). The *Code of Conduct* (NMC, 2018d) sets the standards of conduct, performance and ethics for nurses and midwives and addresses the four domains listed in *Section 9.1*.

### ACTIVITY 9.4

To appreciate how the ethical principles and rules may be useful in guiding decision-making in a contentious situation, reflect on a situation in practice which you were uncertain about or felt uncomfortable about. Use the ethical principles to guide your understanding of this. Then consider how the NMC *Code of Conduct* (ethical rules) may assist in guiding your decision around your actions.

When considering this activity, you will have begun to identify what is influencing your decision-making and whether this is a rational argument based on evidence or an emotional argument based on feelings. A worked example is provided below:

> **WORKED EXAMPLE**
>
> You are currently participating in a vaccination programme for pre-school children. The vaccination clinic is only offered between 9am and 11am on two weekday mornings. In the clinic that you participated in, one child had a severe reaction to the vaccine given. In applying the ethical principles you may consider the following:
>
> *Autonomy* – is respect shown to the individual parents who cannot, or choose not to, participate in the vaccination programme?
>
> *Justice* – does the limited availability of the vaccination programme mean that access is fair for everyone?
>
> *To do good* – does this vaccination programme benefit everyone, does the community benefit from this more than focusing on an individual benefit?
>
> *To do no harm* – has this principle been upheld when there is a severe reaction to a vaccination?

Tannahill (2008) suggests that in many situations there is lack of evidence for the effectiveness of health improvement initiatives, particularly in cross-cutting themes such as dealing with socio-economic inequalities or other diverse equality settings. Tannahill (2008), in recognising these situations where there is a dearth of available evidence, recommends utilising a wider approach to decision-making by those involved in health promotion and improvement which considers ethical principles more explicitly. Decisions on how to proceed are filtered through ethical principles and considered alongside any theoretical or evidence-based knowledge, rather than wholly relying on weak evidence/theory. Therefore, decisions consider such points as social justice and doing no harm first; this offers a balanced and evidence-based approach to health promotion.

## 9.4 Nurses as health promoters and role models

Nurses are perceived as being role models in terms of engaging in good and healthy behaviour; for example, not smoking, maintaining a healthy weight and engaging in exercise (Kemppainen *et al.*, 2013). Although this is not explicitly stated in the educational standards for nursing, there is a shift of perspective occurring. The NMC standards of proficiency (NMC, 2018a, 2018b) are promoting a shift of nurses' knowledge and understanding away from the individual biomedical approach to one of developing a critical consciousness in the population. This change will include empowering and using supportive non-judgemental relationships with others. This is further influenced by the *Code of Conduct* (NMC, 2018d) which identifies the need for nurses to demonstrate professionalism in their behaviour, implying that health-promoting behaviours should also be demonstrated.

> **ACTIVITY 9.5**
>
> Explore what health-promoting behaviours you may exhibit. Reflect on your knowledge of health-promoting behaviours and identify what you practise and why you do this.
>
> You may wish to review this resource as reminder of what healthy behaviours are: www.nhs.uk/change4life

You may have identified that as a student your lifestyle is quite sedentary because you are attending the university and focusing on your studies and that on placement you don't do much exercise or eat healthy food due to the shifts and travel you have to do. If your reflection was like this, you may be able to identify personal, financial, organisational factors or a lack of support, which affects your ability to undertake health-promoting behaviours. Alternatively, you may be active and eat well, but again you may be able to consider the factors that enable you to achieve this.

## 9.4.1 Developing personal health literacy

Having health literacy is the first stage of any healthy behaviour. As we saw in *Chapters 1* and *6*, health literacy is concerned with people having the skills (language, literacy and numeracy), knowledge, understanding and confidence to access, understand, evaluate, use and navigate health information and services (Bröder *et al.*, 2017).

In developing our own personal health literacy there is an implicit suggestion that changing health behaviour can only occur at an individual level; as such it does not recognise the wider notion of health promotion which relies on developing wider collective initiatives that also address health inequalities. Consequently, in using this approach health inequalities may not be challenged and individuals accept the 'blame' for their own poor health (PHE, 2015).

> **ACTIVITY 9.6**
>
> To explore your own health literacy skills and how you may use these to promote action in others, reflect on your own health literacy development. Has your role within nursing and your increasing understanding about choice and systems affected how you engage in healthy behaviour?

An example may be as follows:

When you started your nursing course you may have been a smoker and tried to quit but been unsuccessful. However, the following changes may have facilitated you in stopping smoking:

- Through developing your understanding of motivation, you began to apply this to your own motivation to quit smoking.
- You developed your understanding of the effects of smoking on your health and others'.
- You found a friend who also wanted to quit.
- You found it difficult to smoke at both the university and placement areas.

You may have identified that any behaviour change takes time, knowledge and confidence and success often required the support of others or the organisation. You may also realise that your behaviour has changed because you acknowledged the need to develop your own health literacy (biomedical/individual approach to health) but that actually sustaining this activity is supported by the inability to smoke at the university (a socio-environmental approach to health). A combination of strategies therefore worked.

## 9.4.2 Organisational responsibilities

It is clear from the previous example that changing healthy behaviours requires a wider approach than just from the individual. There is a clear connection between the organisation within which the nurse (or student) may work and the nurse's health or ill health and perceived level of wellbeing. Workplaces such as hospitals, clinics and patients' homes are sometimes experienced by nurses as harmful (Whitehead and Irvine, 2010) with stress, long hours, staff problems, poor resources and emotional labour identified as having a burden on the individual (Javadi-Pashaki and Darvishpour, 2019). If there is a positive healthcare environment in the workplace then individuals experience higher levels of workplace health, evidenced by better teamwork and reduced rates of illness and absenteeism (Whitehead, 2006).

> **ACTIVITY 9.7**
>
> To increase your awareness of the wider organisational influence on individual health promotion, identify which organisations that you have either been in placement with or have worked in have offered the following and reflect on how this affected your wellbeing:
> - Pleasant physical environment (e.g. colour scheme, available natural light, hot/cold)
> - Having available resources to be able to undertake required clinical work
> - Respectful relationships in team
> - Social environment with spaces to meet and opportunity to take breaks
> - Health-promoting schemes
> - Respectful leadership
> - Access to healthy food always at reasonable prices

In the above activity, did you notice that where the organisational experience was positive, this had a direct impact upon your wellbeing?

## 9.4.3 Developing a positive working environment

While some may feel that implementing a change to an organisation is too big a task to undertake, this underestimates the notion that nurses are in a prime position to develop positive work environments. This can occur at all levels, beginning with individual actions that promote patient/client engagement. Examples of this include being a positive role model by demonstrating professionalism, effective communication and teamwork, through to leadership of the clinical environment which promotes healthy behaviours such as ensuring regular break times, respectful leadership and opportunities to relax, and finally to being an advocate at board level in the organisation for all of the above.

> **ACTIVITY 9.8**
>
> To enhance your awareness of the potential influence the nurse may have on developing a positive working environment, reflect on what you may be able to influence and why you think this would promote a healthy environment. Examples may include:
> - When you oversee the team, you ensure everyone takes a break
> - Setting up a system for water bottles to be available throughout the shift

## 9.5 The political dimension of health promotion

Nurses can influence political and public opinion and, as previously discussed, having political awareness is an expected proficiency for the future nurse (NMC, 2018a). Politics are associated with governing a country and are often connected with a set of beliefs which underpin activity. Nurses, through health promotion activity, become involved in the political arena as health promotion policies are politically motivated and driven by the values of the government in power at the time of any intervention (Seedhouse, 2004). The connections are often complex but for the purpose of this chapter it is appropriate that you appreciate there is such a connection and that nurses are actors within any intervention which influences health and ill health.

### 9.5.1 Government and policy

Despite the fact that nurses are one of the largest professional bodies working in health, there is proportionally very little input from nurses into the health policies written by government. Therefore, traditional models remain unchallenged, such as the persistence of a biomedical approach to health promotion, with a focus on preventing disease through pharmacological interventions and encouraging individuals to change behaviour. Seedhouse (2004) suggests that the prominence of the biomedical model of health promotion is reflective of a political agenda of individualism; this approach will always preserve the status quo of the country and promote an individualised or conservative approach to health.

Seedhouse (2004) offers the alternative view that if the government has a belief and will for social equality then the health promotion model focuses on addressing social inequality and developing social change to enact this. This approach recognises that people are equal and there is an emphasis on community development and social health promotion, as we saw in *Chapters 3* and *8*.

## ACTIVITY 9.9

To increase your awareness of the current government influence on health promotion policy, identify the latest health policy published by government and consider which political agenda influenced this. For example, you may wish to review the *Long Term Plan* which was published by the Department of Health in 2018 (www.longtermplan.nhs.uk) and identify which health promotion perspective was used: biomedical/behavioural or social health perspective. Do you think there is a link between this and the government of the time? For example, do the aims of the policy reflect the then government's focus?

### 9.5.2 Global health

The politics of health promotion are also at a global level and affect the health of the world. As we saw in *Chapter 4*, one of the main global actors is the WHO which is the agency established by the United Nations. The work of the WHO is to gather epidemiological data (surveillance) and establish global standards on health matters (WHO, 2019).

## ACTIVITY 9.10

To be aware of the resources available on the WHO website for the wider context of global health, review the information at bit.ly/A9-10A

Then review the similar resource for another country from the list at bit.ly/A9-10B

What similarities or differences are there between the two countries? For example, is the German life expectancy at birth the same as that in the UK? Or Slovakia?

The WHO has a primarily advisory role; it is the responsibility of the individual governments or donors to implement its advice to achieve the targets set from a top-down approach. An example of this could occur when either the government invests, or an organisation such as the World Bank or another country lends money to other governments, to improve health development. Therefore, the health status of a country is influenced by the politics of the individual countries rather than the WHO; as such they are influenced by wider global processes inherent within the individual countries or funders who supply the necessary resources (Trueba, 2016).

Countries are defined by the World Bank as being in one of four income categories: high, upper middle, lower middle and low income (World Bank, 2019). This reflects the average income of a country's residents. This classification is an attempt to understand a country's economic strengths and needs. High income countries such as the UK, USA and Australia provide aid to low income countries such as Uganda, Nepal and Afghanistan. This aid, however, can be conditional, with clear targets established by the funding country which are associated with improving health conditions which may benefit the high income country itself; for example, in providing a healthy future migrant workforce.

It is important that key people such as nurses work together to address global health problems, as disease or inequality in one country may affect another country. This is apparent when dealing with communicable diseases such as HIV or coronavirus. Technical and managerial resources may be required which are larger than some lower income countries can afford on their own. Collective action is needed to fill key gaps in knowledge and to encourage government or voluntary agencies to develop health systems, diagnostics or vaccines to address the most urgent of global health issues related to communicable and non-communicable diseases (Skolnik, 2012). Nurses are again perfectly positioned to develop their influence at a global level, with some nurses already beginning to do this. Examples of this are evident by the activity of the International Council of Nurses (ICN) which is an advocate of key global health issues such as promoting the United Nations' seventeen SDGs (UN, 2020).

### ACTIVITY 9.11

To develop your awareness of nursing in a global context and the connection between global health policy and nursing, review this weblink for the ICN: www.icn.ch/who-we-are

The ICN is a federation of more than 130 national nurse associations. Consider what the political role of this organisation is.

Now explore the following link about how the ICN engages with the WHO: bit.ly/A9-11

### KEY LEARNING POINTS

Four key points to take away from *Chapter 9*:
- ☑ There are professional requirements for health promotion, as stated by the NMC in its proficiencies for RNs and nursing associates.
- ☑ Health improvement and health promotion decisions within your nursing practice can be guided by a biomedical ethical framework and supported by the NMC *Code of Conduct*.
- ☑ The nurse is a health promotion role model for patients/clients, other peers, colleagues and organisations.
- ☑ As a nurse, you need to have an awareness of the political nature of the national and global health policies being implemented.

# REFERENCES

Beauchamp, T. and Childress, J. (2013) *Principles of Biomedical Ethics*, 7th edition. Oxford University Press.

Bröder, J., Okan, O., Bauer, U. *et al*. (2017) Health literacy in childhood and youth: a systematic review of definitions and models. *BMC Public Health,* **17:** 361. Available at: https://bmcpublichealth.biomedcentral.com/articles/10.1186/s12889-017-4267-y (accessed 19 May 2020)

HM Government (2018) *Working together to Safeguard Children*. Available at: https://assets.publishing.service.gov.uk/government/uploads/system/uploads/attachment_data/file/779401/Working_Together_to_Safeguard-Children.pdf (accessed 19 May 2020)

Javadi-Pashaki, N. and Darvishpour, A. (2019) Survey of stress and coping strategies to predict the general health of nursing staff. *Journal of Education and Health Promotion,* **8:** 74. DOI: 10.4103/jehp.jehp_355_18

Kemppainen, V., Tossavainen, K. and Turunen, H. (2013) Nurses' roles in health promotion practice: an integrative review. *Health Promotion International,* **28:** 490–501. Available at: https://academic.oup.com/heapro/article/28/4/490/556908 (accessed 19 May 2020)

Nursing and Midwifery Council (2018a) *Future Nurse: standards of proficiency for registered nurses*. Available at: www.nmc.org.uk/standards/standards-for-nurses (accessed 19 May 2020)

Nursing and Midwifery Council (2018b) Standards for *Nursing Associates*. Available at: www.nmc.org.uk/standards/standards-for-nursing-associates/ (accessed 19 May 2020)

Nursing and Midwifery Council (2018c) *Enabling Professionalism in Nursing and Midwifery Practice*. Available at: www.nmc.org.uk/globalassets/sitedocuments/other-publications/enabling-professionalism.pdf (accessed 19 May 2020)

Nursing and Midwifery Council (2018d) *The Code: professional standards of practice and behaviour for nurses, midwives and nursing associates*. NMC. Available at: www.nmc.org.uk/standards/code/ (accessed 19 May 2020)

Public Health England (2015) *Improving Health Literacy to Reduce Health Inequalities*. Available at: https://assets.publishing.service.gov.uk/government/uploads/system/uploads/attachment_data/file/460710/4b_Health_Literacy-Briefing.pdf (accessed 19 May 2020)

Royal College of Nursing (2018) *Adult Safeguarding, Roles and Competencies for Health Care Staff*. Available at: www.rcn.org.uk/professional-development/publications/pub-007069 (accessed 5 July 2020)

Seedhouse, D. (2004) *Health Promotion: philosophy, prejudice and practice*, 2nd edition. Wiley.

Skolnik, R. (2012) *Global Health 101,* 2nd edition. Jones & Bartlett Learning.

Sykes, S. (2014) 'Approaches to promotiong health'. In Wills, J. (ed.) *Fundamentals of Health Promotion for Nurses,* 2nd edition. Wiley-Blackwell.

Tannahill, A. (2008) Beyond evidence–to ethics: a decision-making framework for health promotion, public health and health improvement. *Health Promotion International,* **23(4):** 380–90. DOI: 10.1093/heapro/dan032

Thomson, R. (2010) 'Health promotion: politics, policy and ethics'. In Whitehead, D. and Irvine, F. (eds) *Health Promotion and Health Education in Nursing*. Palgrave Macmillan.

Trueba, M. (2016) 'The global dimensions of health'. In Artaraz, K. and Hill, M. *Global Social Policy: themes, issues and actors.* Palgrave.

United Nations (2020) *Sustainable Development Goals.* Available at: www.un.org/sustainabledevelopment/ (accessed 19 May 2020)

Whitehead, D. (2006) Health promotion in the practice setting: findings from a review of clinical issues. *Worldviews on Evidence-Based Nursing,* **3(4):** 165–84. DOI: org/10.1111/j.1741-6787.2006.00068.x

Whitehead, D. and Irvine, F. (2010) *Health Promotion and Health Education in Nursing: a framework for practice*. Palgrave Macmillan.

World Bank (2019) *New Country Classifications by Income Level: 2019–2020*. Available at: https://blogs.worldbank.org/opendata/new-country-classifications-income-level-2019-2020 (accessed 19 May 2020)

World Health Organization (2019) *About WHO*. Available at: www.who.int/about (accessed 19 May 2020)

# Chapter 10
# Leadership for health promotion

Alison James

> **LEARNING OUTCOMES**
>
> When you have finished this chapter, you should be able to:
>
> **10.1** Discuss why leadership is important for health promotion
>
> **10.2** Outline the key skills for effective leadership
>
> **10.3** Describe approaches to leading change
>
> **10.4** Demonstrate an understanding of health-promoting leadership

## 10.1 Introduction

In considering why leadership is important in health promotion, it is useful to provide a definition. As we have seen in previous chapters, the WHO defines health promotion thus:

*Health promotion enables people to increase control over their own health. It covers a wide range of social and environmental interventions that are designed to benefit and protect individual people's health and quality of life by addressing and preventing the root causes of ill health, not just focusing on treatment and cure.*

(WHO, 2016)

Within this definition there is a key phrase which suggests that effective leadership is a driving force: *"enables people to increase control over their own health"*. As leadership requires vision and direction and is concerned with aligning people and partnerships, building relationships, motivating and empowering, it is possible to see that in order to facilitate this definition, effective leadership is required. Responding to changing populations and changes in health, wellbeing and disease trajectory requires these abilities so that a vision of what challenges may present are anticipated and responded to appropriately.

To understand the role of leadership in health promotion further, it is important to first explore what 'leadership' means. As a student, you will be learning and observing many different approaches to leadership within healthcare. As you gain experience, you will form your own ideas of what it means to you as a professional and what it means within the healthcare context.

This chapter will present some of the key concepts of leadership in health promotion. Thinking of how leadership may influence the delivery of care, as well as how it can influence health promotion in our patients and our colleagues and areas of work, will support your formation of ideas while also enabling you to understand why developing an insight is important.

> **ACTIVITY 10.1**
>
> Identify who you consider to be a leader, in work or in your personal life. Write down the qualities and characteristics that make them a leader.

## 10.2 Defining leadership

Since 1948 the WHO has provided a macro level core leadership role for global health promotion in its functions of:
- leadership in essential areas of need and enabling a partnership approach to tackle those needs
- directing a research programme and motivating the progress and distribution of evidence-based knowledge
- establishing standards for health and evaluating their application
- conveying ethical policy based on evidence
- being agents for change and promoting sustainable programmes
- observing and scrutinising health trends globally.

(WHO, 2014)

While the WHO provides this important element of macro leadership, we also need to consider personal (micro) leadership roles and organisational (meso) leadership in the context of health promotion (*Figure 10.1*).

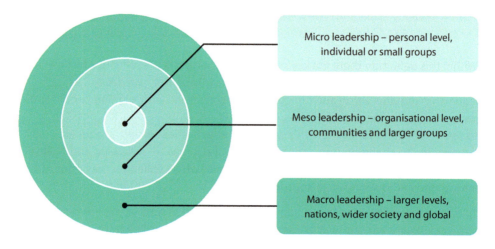

**Figure 10.1** *Levels of leadership in the context of health promotion.*

First, it is necessary to create a definition. Leadership can be defined in many ways and numerous leadership theories have been developed and discussed within the texts; all are relevant and can help you to think about what leadership means to you. However, while these theories provide different approaches to leadership, none provides the absolute definition and solution to what approach works well. Some of these theories are presented in *Figure 10.2*; it will be useful for you to explore sources and texts which provide a further overview of theories and qualities of leadership to provide a broad exploration of defining leadership qualities, such as Jones and Bennett (2018) and Barr and Dowding (2019).

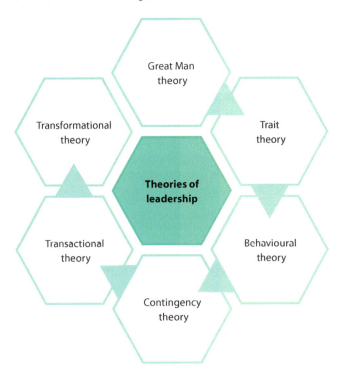

**Figure 10.2** *Examples of leadership theories.*

### ACTIVITY 10.2

Consider the leadership styles in *Figure 10.2* and write down your definition of what leadership is.

Thinking of your own experience of leadership and reading about different theories will help you to identify your own thoughts of what it means to you and allow you to think of where you apply leadership skills. Burns (2010) presents leadership as two different types: transactional and transformational. Transactional leaders focus on standards, targets, goals and performance, with penalties for not achieving these. An example of this approach within healthcare is provided by Barr and Dowding (2019) as the 4-hour rule for waiting in Accident and Emergency.

Transformational leaders act in the interests of the team or followers by responding to a need through positive change, having a vision for change and engaging the team in the vision (Barr and Dowding, 2019). It is also important to understand that more than one approach can be used and there are times when one may be more effective in gaining the best outcome. For example, a transactional approach may be more effective when targets for improvements in health are urgent; for example, the Ebola crisis needed urgent action with stringent measures for preventing and minimising spread. However, a transformational approach may be more effective in implementing a change over a long period within a team, by agreeing a vision and engaging all in the process. For example, when there is a local policy change which needs to be implemented in a multidisciplinary clinical area, an engaging transformational style would ensure the team take ownership by having a shared vision. Leadership skills are needed in healthcare and nursing to ensure that the main vision and aspiration of the organisation and those that work within it are achieved; to deliver safe and effective patient care to maximum effect, despite the challenges.

Defining an approach to leadership can be helpful for you as it will impact your approach to clinical practice as you progress in your career. This is important for leading health promotion initiatives and providing influence in improving health and preventing disease.

### ACTIVITY 10.3

Think about the differences between transactional and transformational leadership, as defined above. Which do you think is more aligned to your values and approach to nursing?

Recent development of leadership theory includes 'compassionate leadership', 'values-based leadership' and 'congruent leadership'. West *et al.* (2017) describe compassionate leadership as aligning well to healthcare, as it approaches leadership as an open, non-blaming, collective style. Congruent leadership is defined by Stanley (2019) as the actions of the leader being compatible with their values and beliefs. Guided by commitment and compassion, congruent leaders have a high regard for others, establish strong relationships and are values-driven (Stanley, 2019). Both approaches to leadership break from the more traditional styles from industry and business, such as those shown in *Figure 10.2*, and are well situated within health as they reflect the elements of professional practice in basing decisions on evidence and taking a caring, helping and empathetic approach (James, 2019).

### ACTIVITY 10.4

Consider *Figure 10.3* and reflect on how the elements of compassionate and congruent leadership fit with the professional values, beliefs and standards within health promotion, as set out by the *Code* (Nursing and Midwifery Council, 2018).

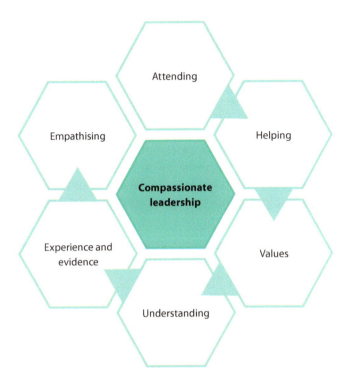

**Figure 10.3** *Key elements of compassionate and congruent leadership. Adapted from James (2019).*

Thinking further about your own leadership style from different perspectives may help you to become more self-aware. For example, in *Activity 10.1*, what were the qualities and characteristics you noted down? Do you have any of these characteristics? Do you think these are essential or are there other characteristics that you have which are equally important for good leadership? This can be considered as getting to know your own 'traits' or characteristics of leadership.

Other aspects which may be useful for you to consider are:
- How important is someone's position in an organisation for leadership?
- Is leadership a process rather than a quality or position?
- Are leaders always considered powerful?

### ACTIVITY 10.5

Considering the questions above and your own role and professional practice, do you think you can be a leader in your current position? What are the challenges and how might you overcome these to influence your own practice and that of others?

## 10.3 Self-awareness and emotional intelligence

Being aware of your own personal skills, your own emotions and how you respond to others is known as emotional intelligence (EI) (Goleman, 1996). As we saw in *Chapter 7*, having EI means that a person is aware of how knowledge and emotions influence the way in which decisions are made and how a person responds and acts. Having high EI, self-awareness and awareness for others means a person recognises their own and others' emotional reactions. They can respond to people empathetically, while taking a positive, respectful and problem-solving approach to the situation (Barr and Dowding, 2019). This is important for all nursing professionals and for effective leadership as it promotes respect and honesty and ensures we are considering others' emotional situations, which may affect the way they act or behave, while also being aware of our own emotions and how we respond. EI can be applied to interactions and relationships with patients, team members and other staff, as it allows you to consider the whole context of an interaction and what the most positive and suitable response may be to promote good relationships and outcomes.

To understand and develop self-awareness, a model such as the Johari window (Luft, 1969) could be used, as seen in *Chapter 7*. This model (*Figure 10.4*) allows exploration of four areas: the open, the blind, the hidden and the unknown. Jones and Bennett helpfully describe the areas as follows:

> *The open area is the area that we know about ourselves and that others also know about us. Examples may be physical characteristics and personality traits.*
>
> *The blind area is made up of characteristics that others know about us, but we are not aware of. This may include communication skills that others are aware of, but we have no insight into.*
>
> *The hidden area is made up of things we know about ourselves that we wish to keep private.*
>
> *The unknown area is unknown to both ourselves and others.*
>
> (Jones and Bennett, 2018, pp. 41–2)

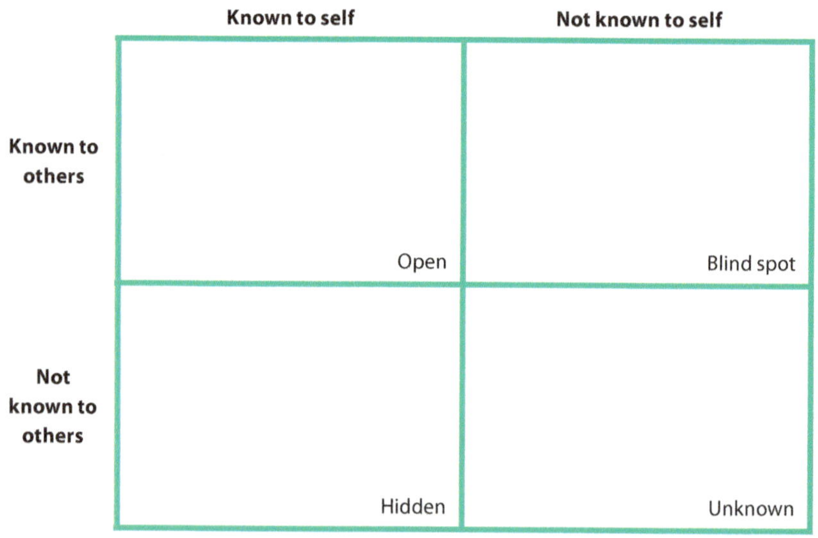

|  | Known to self | Not known to self |
|---|---|---|
| **Known to others** | Open | Blind spot |
| **Not known to others** | Hidden | Unknown |

**Figure 10.4** *The Johari window (Luft, 1969).*

### ACTIVITY 10.6

Use the Johari window to describe your characteristics in each area. Consider how you may decrease the size of the blind spot area by seeking others' views of your traits.

Another way you can become more self-aware is through reflection and keeping reflective diaries. As this forms part of our professional requirements by the Nursing and Midwifery Council, this can be an effective way of exploring your EI and self-awareness, as your experience as a professional nurse develops and extends.

## 10.4 Emotional intelligence and health promotion

Public health and health promotion are concerned with enhancing quality of life and health within populations. Understanding emotions and responses to health and lifestyle can allow nurses to design and effect the best outcomes for people by providing insight into why choices are made. Here, examples of research are provided such as Bhochhibhoya and Branscum (2015) who consider the importance of EI and how health promotion may be approached. They suggest that working with adolescents and young adults on developing self-awareness and EI may contribute to their lifestyle choices and therefore longer-term health outcomes. Further research is needed in this area which may support insight into how EI could be used within health promotion as a preventative approach.

### 10.4.1 Smoking

Smoking tobacco and the associated preventable conditions of lung disease, cardiovascular disease and cancer are a public health issue and adolescents are a vulnerable population due to peer pressure and tobacco advertising. Trinidad and Johnson (2002) explored the relationship between EI and adolescent smoking and drinking alcohol in 205 adolescents in southern California. Using an EI measuring scale, an association between smoking and low EI in adolescents in the 7th and 8th grade found they were twice as likely to be involved in smoking than those students with higher EI.

### 10.4.2 Negative lifestyle behaviours

Brackett, Mayer and Warner (2004) found low EI to be a predictor of negative life outcomes. The researchers explored 330 students' self-care behaviour, leisure activity and interpersonal relationships. Female students measured higher levels of EI, and lower EI in male students was associated with negative lifestyle outcomes which included illegal drug use, alcohol use and reduced peer relationships. The researchers suggest low EI to be associated with negative behaviours for male higher education students.

### 10.4.3 EI in nursing

The concepts that comprise EI have been acknowledged as important in relation to leadership in healthcare professions; ensuring challenges are confronted and provision of appropriate and effective service provision is led with consideration (Carragher and Gormley, 2016; Akerjordet and Severinsson, 2008). Furthermore, evidence suggests developing EI in undergraduate nursing students to enhance future leadership strengths is needed. In public health, this would enable a caring, compassionate and values-based approach to leading healthcare delivery and health promotion (Codier *et al.*, 2010; Duygulu, Hiçdurmaz and Akyar, 2011; Benson *et al.*, 2012; Foster *et al.*, 2015).

> **ACTIVITY 10.7**
>
> Think of a situation where you have been involved in, or witnessed, a challenging interaction in a health promotion activity, either with a colleague or between a professional and a patient. Think about the situation from both sides. How did those involved respond and do you think they considered each other's emotions?
>
> Reflect on how this may have been different if both had applied consideration of the other's experience.

## 10.5 Leadership skills in practice

In your experience as a student and when you qualify, you will develop skills which all include aspects of leadership, for example:
- planning and organising the provision of care
- making decisions
- working effectively within teams
- communicating clearly
- planning and implementing change
- evaluating care.

> **ACTIVITY 10.8**
>
> The list above is relevant to all aspects of leadership and all areas of healthcare. Reflect on how you think these are important to health promotion. For example, you may want to consider how you would use your leadership style in planning a health promotion project. Who would you need to engage with and who would be involved in making decisions? In terms of working within the team, do you know the strengths and characteristics of the team and would you consider allocating certain tasks to some? If so, why? How would you know if your project is successful – what would you need to measure and when?

## 10.6 Leadership or management?

It is useful to further define your view of your own leadership competencies by considering the differences between management and leadership. Management can be defined as a more functional activity and role which involves setting goals, allocating resources, generating solutions and ensuring targets and aims are met. The managerial role is usually hierarchical and takes a transactional approach to ensure the organisation functions in its parts.

Leaders, however, tend to influence rather than direct; they have a broader view of the end vision and consider the relationships needed to achieve this. In health promotion this distinction is important as we see from the WHO (2016) definition at the beginning of this chapter; it is concerned with having an overall view of the aim and goal for a wider population and considering how to achieve that. A useful way to differentiate between leadership and management is to consider management as **analysis**, the separation of issues into different parts or tasks, and leadership as **synthesis**, the combination of factors to provide a combined vision (Porter-O'Grady and Malloch, 2016). In the context of health promotion, while management is also important to deliver appropriate activities and functions, leadership sets the extended course for improving the health of a population.

### ACTIVITY 10.9

Consider the elements of management and leadership below. Reflect on your experience of management and leadership and how these activities fit or overlap between both. Using the overlapping circles in *Figure 10.5*, plot these elements and consider how some may overlap.

**Management**
Organising staffing
Managing budgets
Developing solutions
Allocating tasks and roles
Organising workload
Risk averse
Coordinating activities
Ensuring targets are met

**Leadership**
Communicating aims and goals
Inspiring teams
Providing the vision
Empowering individuals
Motivating change
Accepting risk
Establishing strategic direction
Influencing stakeholders

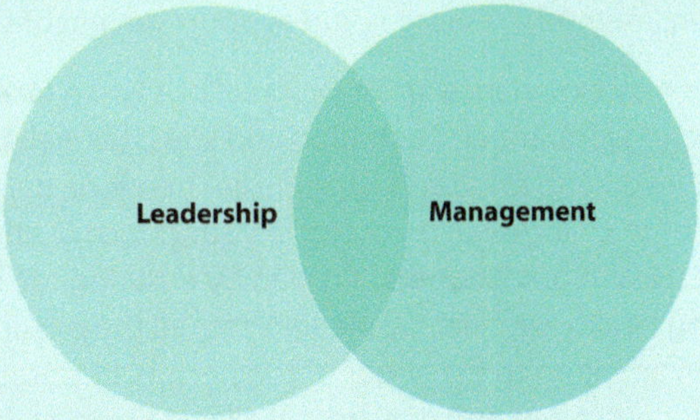

**Figure 10.5** *Interrelationship between leadership and management.*

## 10.7 Leading for change

Change is a constant in healthcare; whether it is due to an increasing ageing population, the prevalence of disease or the effects of global warming (WHO, 2018). Promoting health and wellbeing within populations requires an ability to adapt and respond to the challenges of implementing change. Leaders are channels for implementing change and for driving agendas for change and responding to anticipated demands. As countries become increasingly connected and interdependent with moving workforces, leading change presents further challenges; issues such as the culture, beliefs and values of all populations need to be considered, as well as equality of provision of healthcare. Globalisation has given many opportunities for sharing practice, supporting innovation in research and healthcare; however, it also produces challenges.

> **ACTIVITY 10.10**
>
> Consider your response to change in practice. How do you usually feel when a new way of working is introduced? Do you respond positively? Write down the negative and positive feelings you have about changes in your working practice. Think of others in your team – do they respond well to change?

In undertaking *Activity 10.10* you may have noticed that people respond differently to change. Being prepared for how people respond is an important part of leadership, as there are methods to manage this and ensure the team can move into the new way or approach needed, to ensure the vision of change is achieved. Kotter and Schlesinger (1979) set out four reasons for resisting change:

- self-interest – people may feel the change is not helpful or beneficial for them
- lack of trust or misunderstanding
- people prefer stability and security
- different expectations.

Being aware of these issues can allow a leader to prepare the team by providing clear communication of the reasons for change and the evidence for making the change. In health promotion, this may need further planning as it may involve addressing large populations in making lifestyle changes. Empowering people to enable them to take control of their health is a key role in health promotion; providing people with the information, methods, resources and support can enable change to occur.

It is possible people may experience an array of feelings when faced with changes to their lifestyle, such as loss, anger, frustration and stress, as well as more positive feelings such as achievement, pride and happiness. Therefore, being aware of possible responses to change can be useful in your choice of approach and leading the change. Health practitioners can lead by ensuring the message and reason for improving health are clear, by planning for all the possible responses and being flexible in adapting to the needs of the person. Imposed change can result in unsuccessful outcomes and may be less likely to be sustained, so careful consideration of how a change is to be introduced is important, as we have seen in

*Chapter 2*. Barr and Dowding (2019) set out the possible effects of a change that is imposed, including:
- feelings of anxiety and uncertainty
- lack of control
- lack of understanding
- resistance
- uncertain commitment.

These effects are the opposite to enabling empowerment; so when leading change, it may be helpful to adopt strategies suggested by Kotter and Schlesinger (1979) such as:
- educating and persuading
- including and involving
- supporting and enabling
- negotiating
- influencing
- reviewing at each stage
- responding appropriately
- being creative in seeking out alternative approaches
- providing the evidence base for change.

### ACTIVITY 10.11

Think of a successful health promotion campaign. Why do you think it went well? Were any of the above strategies used?

Examples may be found on the following websites:
**Public Health England**: bit.ly/A10-11A
**Public Health Wales**: bit.ly/A10-11B
**Public Health Scotland**: bit.ly/A10-11C
**Public Health Agency Northern Ireland**: bit.ly/A10-11D

## 10.8 Planning, implementing and evaluating

In health promotion, it is necessary to consider the impact of the proposed change, as well as considering how it can be sustained. It is useful to consider the strengths and drivers which can support the implementation of the change. Lewin's (1951) force field analysis is a useful tool to support the planning, implementation and evaluation of sustainability. Using qualitative (soft) and quantitative (hard) information, it is possible to use the tool to plan the impact of the change and consider its positive driving forces and negative resisting forces, in order to provide a possible estimated prediction of success. This is also a useful tool as it can be used with all stakeholders; the team, service users and patients, to engage all in the planning and process of implementing change, encouraging commitment and empowering those involved.

One example of using a force field analysis to plot the driving forces and resisting forces might be for increasing activity in those aged over 65 years in a rural area. Driving forces may be improving social contact for isolated people, enhanced wellbeing, improved health and reduced aches and pains. Resisting forces may be difficulty in reaching the meeting point due to lack of transport, lack of confidence, lack of knowledge about health benefits and mobility issues. By plotting the forces using different sized arrows to indicate the strength of the influence, it is possible to view which forces are stronger (*Figure 10.6*). Consider how established and immovable those strong forces are, which forces can be influenced to overcome the challenges, and what strategies need to be implemented to take the plan forward.

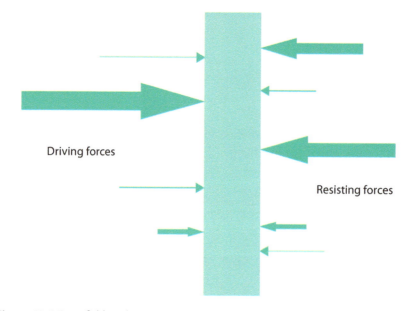

**Figure 10.6** *Force field analysis.*

### ACTIVITY 10.12

Using *Figure 10.6*, think of a small change you would like to make personally or in practice. Plot the forces and consider your approach to taking the change forward.

A shared decision-making approach to health promotion may be adopted more widely and in strategic public health directions, for example as seen in the prudent healthcare policy in Wales (Bevan Commission, 2013). Within this policy, prudent healthcare aims to provide patients and the public with an equal partnership with the healthcare professionals in making decisions about their treatment and care, as well as shaping future health services. This can enable leadership to be shared also, by professionals and all stakeholders, taking a collaborative approach to leading change. This approach can also encourage sustainability and build capacity, as investment in the programme by those at whom it is aimed can result in a commitment and engagement in its success.

## 10.9 Health-promoting leadership

While we have discussed the importance of leadership in health promotion, there is a further aspect of leadership which relates to the work environment and culture of our organisations, which needs consideration. Staffing shortages, pressures of the demand of workload and maintaining the quality of care provision we want to provide, mean mastery in nursing leadership is important to support and drive forward professional integrity. Being able to lead in maintaining and nurturing a healthy supportive collegiate workplace is the responsibility of all nurses to ensure we are effective and maintain high standards of care. Akerjordet, Furunes and Haver (2018) suggest strong leadership within nursing can encourage increased satisfaction in the workplace, decrease costs and promote high quality nursing care. Ensuring the organisation promotes a culture of health and wellbeing may encourage a valued and motivated workforce.

> 'Health-promoting leadership concerns creating a culture for health-promoting workplaces and values that inspire and motivate employees to participate in such a development.'
>
> (Eriksson, Axelsson and Axelsson, 2011, p. 17)

This applies across the healthcare professions to ensure optimum patient outcomes and effective teamworking. While nurses try to provide high quality care for patients and service users, there is sometimes a tendency to place personal health and wellbeing as a lower priority. Evidence from research demonstrates high rates of burnout and negative health outcomes in nurses where workplace empowerment is lacking (Laschinger, Wong and Grau, 2013). There is, therefore, a place for health-promoting leadership to ensure responsibility is acknowledged for the workforce's wellbeing, recognising the feelings and needs of colleagues and peers within the workplace. A health-focused and motivating work environment is essential if nursing is to flourish and nursing leadership at all levels can encourage this holistic approach.

An integrative review by Akerjordet, Furunes and Haver (2018) of research into health-promoting leadership found attributes of a health-promoting leader in nursing requires:
- courage and responsibility
- a holistic view of leadership
- an approach to enhance recovery and reduce stress
- acknowledgement of the context of the organisation.

### ACTIVITY 10.13

Consider your own work environment and colleagues. Is there an emphasis on health and wellbeing for staff? Reflecting on your leadership skills, what could you do to make improvements in how staff wellbeing is considered?

> **KEY LEARNING POINTS**
>
> Three key points to take away from *Chapter 10*:
> - ✅ Defining an approach to leadership can be helpful for you as it will impact on your approach to clinical practice as you progress in your health promotion role.
> - ✅ EI is important for all nursing professionals and for effective leadership, as it promotes respect and honesty and ensures consideration of others' emotional situations.
> - ✅ Leaders are channels for implementing change and for driving agendas for change, responding to anticipated demands; planning and anticipating responses to change is a useful strategy.

# REFERENCES

Akerjordet, K. and Severinsson, E. (2008) Emotionally intelligent nurse leadership: a literature review study. *Journal of Nursing Management*, **16:** 565–77.

Akerjordet, K., Furunes, T. and Haver, A. (2018) Health-promoting leadership: an integrative review and future research agenda. *Journal of Advanced Nursing*, **74(7):** 1505–16. DOI: 10.1111/jan.13567.

Barr, J. and Dowding, L. (2019) *Leadership in Healthcare*, 4th edition. SAGE.

Benson, G., Martin, L., Ploeg, J. and Wessel, J. (2012) Longitudinal study of emotional intelligence, leadership and caring in undergraduate nursing students. *Journal of Nursing Education*, **51(2):** 95–101.

Bevan Commission (2013) *Prudent Healthcare Principles*. Available at: www.bevancommission.org/en/prudent-healthcare (accessed 19 May 2020)

Bhochhibhoya, A. and Branscum, P. (2015) Emotional intelligence: a place in public health promotion and education. *Paediatrics and Health*, **3:** 2. Available at: www.academia.edu/12342522/Emotional_intelligence_a_place_in_public_health_promotion_and_education (accessed 19 May 2020)

Brackett, M., Mayer, J. and Warner, R. (2004) Emotional intelligence and its relation to everyday behaviour. *Personality and Individual Differences*, **36:** 1387–1402. DOI: doi:10.1016/S0191-8869(03)00236-8

Burns, J. (2010) *Leadership*. Harper Perennial Modern Classics.

Carragher, J. and Gormley, K. (2016) Leadership and emotional intelligence in nursing and midwifery education and practice: a discussion paper. *Journal of Advanced Nursing*, **73(1):** 85–96. DOI: 10.1111/jan.13141

Codier, E., Muneno, L., Franey, K. and Matsuura, F. (2010) Is emotional intelligence an important concept for nursing practice? *Journal of Psychiatric and Mental Health Nursing*, **17(10):** 940–8.

Duygulu, S., Hiçdurmaz, D. and Akyar, I. (2011) Nursing students' leadership and emotional intelligence in Turkey. *Journal of Nursing Education*, **50(5):** 281–5.

Eriksson, A., Axelsson, R. and Axelsson, S. (2011) Health promoting leadership – different views of the concept. *Work*, **40(1):** 75–84. DOI: 10.3233/WOR-2011-1208

Foster, K., McCloughen, A., Delgado, C., Kefalas, C. and Harkness, E. (2015) Emotional intelligence education in pre-registration nursing programmes: an integrative review. *Nurse Education Today*, **35(3):** 510–17.

Goleman, D. (1996) *Emotional Intelligence: why it can matter more than IQ*. Bloomsbury.

James, A. (2019) 'Compassionate leadership'. In Clouston, T. *et al. Becoming a Caring and Compassionate Practitioner*. Available at: https://caringpractitioner.co.uk/index.php/compassionate-leadership/ (accessed 19 May 2020)

Jones, L. and Bennett, C. (2018) *Leadership: for nursing, health and social care students*. Lantern Publishing.

Kotter, J. and Schlesinger, L. (1979) *Choosing Strategies for Change*. Harvard Business Review. Available at: https://hbr.org/2008/07/choosing-strategies-for-change (accessed 19 May 2020)

Laschinger, H., Wong, C. and Grau, A. (2013) Authentic leadership, empowerment and burnout: a comparison in new graduates and experienced nurses. *Journal of Nursing Management*, **21(3):** 541–52. DOI: 10.1111/j.1365-2834.2012.0137

Lewin, K. (1951) *Field Theory in Social Sciences: selected theoretical papers*. Harper.

Luft, J. (1969) *Of Human Interaction*. National Press.

Nursing and Midwifery Council (2018) *The Code: professional standards of practice and behaviour for nurses, midwives and nursing associates*. NMC. Available at www.nmc.org.uk/standards/code/ (accessed 19 May 2020)

Porter-O'Grady, T. and Malloch, K. (2016) *Leadership in Nursing Practice: changing the landscape of health care*. Jones and Bartlett Learning.

Stanley, D. (2019) *Values-Based Leadership in Healthcare: congruent leadership explored*. SAGE.

Trinidad, D. and Johnson, C. (2002) The association between emotional intelligence and early adolescent tobacco and alcohol use. *Personality and Individual Differences*, **32:** 95–105. DOI:org/10.1016/S0191-8869(01)00008-3

West, M., Eckert, R., Collins, B. and Chowla, R. (2017*) Caring to Change: how compassionate leadership can stimulate innovation in health care*. King's Fund. Available at: www.kingsfund.org.uk/publications/caring-change (accessed 19 May 2020)

World Health Organization (2014) *Not Merely the Absence of Disease*. Twelfth General programme of Work. Available at www.who.int/about/resources_planning/twelfth-gpw/en/ (accessed 19 May 2020)

World Health Organization (2016) *What is Health Promotion?* Available at: www.who.int/features/qa/health-promotion/en/ (accessed 19 May 2020)

World Health Organization (2018) *Climate Change and Health*. Available at: www.who.int/news-room/fact-sheets/detail/climate-change-and-health (accessed 19 May 2020)°

# Chapter 11
# Evidence-based health promotion

Judith Carrier

> **LEARNING OUTCOMES**
>
> When you have finished this chapter, you should be able to:
>
> 11.1 Define evidence-based healthcare and understand the historical origin of the term
>
> 11.2 Outline what constitutes evidence in healthcare practice and how this compares to health promotion
>
> 11.3 Discuss the umbrella term 'evidence synthesis'
>
> 11.4 Debate what works when applying evidence to healthcare practice and identify some of the difficulties in implementing evidence
>
> 11.5 Describe how evidence can be applied to health promotion activities.

## 11.1 Introduction

In this chapter we consider the historical roots of the term evidence-based practice (EBP), including the original derivation of the term from the evidence-based medicine (EBM) movement, what EBP means to today's health practitioners, the skills required to implement evidence-based healthcare (EBHC) and how evidence can be applied to health promotion activities.

Knowing the evidence base is not enough to change practice. Lizarondo and McArthur (2017) note that to achieve facilitated change requires:

> … *effective leadership and facilitation skills, including the ability to articulate a plan and a purpose; inform, motivate and persuade others; solicit support; and foster team development.*
>
> (Lizarondo and McArthur, 2017, p. 459)

This is equally applicable to health promotion activities as to any other clinical activity you undertake.

> **ACTIVITY 11.1**
>
> Consider how the scientific principles of EBP apply to healthcare practice today.
>
> You will need to refer to the three critical elements of EBP: evidence from research, clinical expertise and client/patient preference. Think how these can be applied to the health promotion activities you are involved in within your practice.

## 11.2 Defining evidence-based healthcare

Where does the term evidence-based healthcare come from and how can this term be applied to health promotion policies and activities? The ideas underpinning EBP are certainly not new, indeed Glasziou (2011) argues that they have been evolving for centuries, with roots in psychology, sociology and philosophy. The underlying principles of EBP, which included locating, appraising and using research and systematic and scientific principles to help clinicians make decisions based on the best information available, were developed in the 1980s, in the Department of Clinical Epidemiology and Biostatistics at McMaster University in Canada (Evidence-Based Medicine Working Group, 1992). The term 'evidence-based medicine', from which EBP and later on the term EBHC was derived, was first proposed in the 1990s by Gordon Guyatt, the leader of an international group of clinicians formed to consider results of recent research when treating patients, the initial focus being on doctors making decisions at the bedside of patients (Glasziou, 2011). The term first appeared in print as follows:

> *A NEW paradigm for medical practice is emerging. Evidence based medicine de-emphasizes intuition, unsystematic clinical experience, and pathophysiologic rationale as sufficient grounds for clinical decision-making and stresses the examination of evidence from clinical research.*
>
> (Evidence-Based Medicine Working Group, 1992, p. 2420)

Since these early definitions EBHC has grown and evolved, along with the appreciation that while research is important for healthcare activities, EBHC includes several components, of which research is only one. One area that has evolved from EBHC is evidence-based health promotion. However, when considering evidence-based health promotion Rychetnik and Wise (2004) argue that many policies are not supported by high quality evidence and the greatest challenge for those implementing health promotion interventions is when they identify health promotion goals with an evident need where evidence is weak or non-existent.

A simpler definition of evidence-based healthcare that fits well with health promotion activities is supplied by Hicks (1997):

> *Evidence based health care takes place when decisions that affect the care of patients are taken with due weight accorded to all valid, relevant information.*
>
> (Hicks, 1997, p. 321)

Hicks (1997) explains this further by saying that there are many factors that influence the decisions we make about the care of patients/clients. This includes patient preferences and availability of resources as well as evidence from research. As long as we appraise this information and give it 'due weight' then we should not make a decision on only one sort of evidence.

For example, suppose you read a research study that showed there was strong evidence that attending a regular group exercise class is the best way to reduce the risk of cardiovascular disease. However, your patient/client lives in a remote area where classes are not available or prefers to exercise alone. In this instance you may need to consider another approach that may not have the same research evidence to support it, but is more appropriate for the particular patient/client.

### ACTIVITY 11.2

Think of health promotion activities you have observed or been involved in. What do you know about the evidence base for these interventions?

## 11.3 What is evidence?

We hear a lot about evidence in healthcare, but what exactly does the word 'evidence' mean and how can it help us in practice? The Cambridge Dictionary (2019a) defines evidence as a noun meaning *"anything that helps to prove that something is or is not true"*.

'Evidence-based' is further defined as an adjective that means *"supported by a large amount of scientific research"* (Cambridge Dictionary, 2019b). However, as we noted earlier when considering healthcare, lots of different things impact on the decisions we make about patient/client care and while scientific research is important, there may be other personal, contextual and economic influences you need to consider.

The WHO (2019) *Global Programme on Health Promotion Effectiveness* states that we need evidence for health promotion in order to:
- identify the best possible ways to promote health
- make decisions for policy development and funding allocation
- demonstrate to decision makers that health promotion works and is an effective strategy in public health
- support practitioners in project development and evaluation
- show the wider community the benefits of health promotion actions
- advocate for health promotion development.

(WHO, 2019)

In health promotion, research evidence can include all types of studies, both quantitative studies that measure the effects of a health promotion intervention, determining whether it works (for example a dietary, lifestyle or behavioural activity) and qualitative studies that consider how and why activities work, what people think about them and what makes people comply (or not comply) with health promotion advice or activities.

Studies that draw on quantitative data (numbers) include:
- randomised controlled trials
- quasi-experimental studies
- cohort studies
- case control studies
- descriptive observational studies.

Studies that draw on qualitative data (narrative words and text) include:
- ethnography
- phenomenology
- grounded theory
- qualitative descriptive studies.

Evidence can also include secondary sources of evidence such as clinical guidelines, systematic reviews (summaries of evidence) and policy documents (although policy documents may not always be evidence-based). Local guidance should be created from an established evidence base that draws upon a systematic search and appraisal of relevant literature.

In the last decade an approach to reviewing and synthesising evidence, known as realist synthesis, has become more popular in order to understand why complex interventions, such as health promotion, work or don't work. A realist synthesis asks 'what works, for whom and in what circumstances?' and attempts to understand not only what interventions are effective, but investigates the mechanism behind this. This is particularly pertinent to health promotion where we might be interested not only in whether something works, but whether it requires certain conditions to make it work. For further reading see Rycroft-Malone *et al.* (2012).

### ACTIVITY 11.3

Based on all that you have learnt in the previous chapters, make a list of all the things that can determine whether a health promotion activity works (or not), including human and resource factors. What type of evidence would have helped you in selecting the right approach?

For example, if you want to know whether something worked or not, you will need to draw on studies using quantitative data; if you want to know how someone feels about an intervention then you will draw on studies using qualitative data.

### ACTIVITY 11.4

Make a list of databases where you could search for research evidence to support health promotion activities.

These can be found on your university website, and/or through an Athens subscription if you are employed by the NHS, or RCN webpages. Availability will vary but typical databases you could search include: TRIP, MEDLINE, CINAHL, PsycINFO, Scopus, Web of Science, ASSIA. Ask your local librarian for further support.

## 11.4 Systematic reviews/evidence synthesis

### 11.4.1 Evidence synthesis

Evidence synthesis is an umbrella term for information that has been brought together from a range of sources to help practitioners make decisions. Evidence syntheses are sometimes called 'secondary evidence' as they bring together, appraise and evaluate data that has been obtained from other sources. This could be from primary research studies such as those listed earlier or could be a gathering of information and knowledge from various sources, including experts in the field. The essential criteria of an evidence synthesis are that it should be honest, assess the included evidence for any bias and be succinct for decision-makers to read.

The journal *Nature*, considered one of the world's leading scientific journals, produced a set of four principles for evidence synthesis that it recommends should be adhered to by those who commission, write and use evidence syntheses: they should be inclusive, rigorous, transparent and accessible (Donnelly *et al.*, 2018).

> **ACTIVITY 11.5**
>
> Read the article by Donnelly *et al.* (2018) at bit.ly/A11-5 and make brief notes in the columns below related to what the article says about each of the four principles.

| | |
|---|---|
| Inclusive | |
| Rigorous | |
| Transparent | |
| Accessible | |

Other types of evidence syntheses you will come across include systematic reviews, rapid reviews, umbrella reviews and clinical guidelines. The key to judging the quality of evidence syntheses is that you should be able to see how the authors sourced the evidence that informed the synthesis, how they determined what evidence should be included, how they appraised this evidence to eliminate bias and how this information is combined. Whether it is readable and easily accessible are additional important criteria.

## 11.4.2 Systematic reviews

Systematic reviews are a particular form of evidence synthesis that bring together and summarise data from primary research studies. They can involve a team of researchers and should be transparent throughout about the methods they use to search for the literature, select studies in terms of their ability to answer the research question, appraise studies to assess the methodological quality and how they analyse and synthesise the data from these studies to make recommendations for practice or future research. All systematic reviews should be preceded by publication of a plan, called a protocol, that sets out how the review will be conducted.

Guidance on reporting and publishing systematic reviews is available from the Preferred Reporting Items for Systematic Reviews and Meta-Analyses (PRISMA) website: www.prisma-statement.org.

There are several databases and journals that specialise in publishing systematic reviews and/or protocols and teaching systematic review methods; *Table 11.1* shows some of these.

**Table 11.1** *Databases and journals specialising in systematic reviews*

| Name | Website |
|---|---|
| The Cochrane Database of Systematic Reviews | www.cochranelibrary.com/cdsr/about-cdsr |
| Campbell Collaboration | https://campbellcollaboration.org/ |
| JBI Database of Systematic Reviews and Implementation Reports | https://joannabriggs.org/ebp#database |
| BMC Systematic Reviews | https://systematicreviewsjournal.biomedcentral.com/ |
| Centre for Reviews and Dissemination, University of York | www.york.ac.uk/crd/ |
| ScHARR, University of Sheffield | www.sheffield.ac.uk/scharr/sections/heds/sys_rev |
| EPPI-Centre | https://eppi.ioe.ac.uk/cms/ |
| PROSPERO (protocols) | www.crd.york.ac.uk/PROSPERO/ |

Not all systematic reviews will be published in a specialised systematic review database or journal. Authors may sometimes prefer to publish systematic reviews in a journal aimed at a specific group of healthcare professions, for example nurses. If you are searching for systematic reviews, search the databases you have listed in *Activity 11.4* to make sure you have not missed anything; you can apply a filter to the search to make it more specific to systematic reviews.

### ACTIVITY 11.6

Search for 'health promotion' in the TRIP database www.tripdatabase.com using the search facility and see how many systematic reviews you can find.

Once you have found them refine your search to 'health promotion carer' and see how many systematic reviews you can find through this search.

Clue: Look at the right-hand side of the database after you have searched for evidence type and you will see a category called systematic reviews.

Evidence synthesis and systematic reviews are not limited to healthcare; they include a wide range of topics such as education, crime and justice, social welfare and international development.

### ACTIVITY 11.7

Use the What Works Network (2018) at bit.ly/A11-7 and make a list of the topic areas covered.

## 11.5 Applying evidence to practice – what works?

So how do we know what works and what doesn't? Hopefully the preceding part of this chapter will have started to make you think about how we evaluate health promotion activities and then act on recommendations, rather than just developing activities ad hoc, without giving proper thought and attention to whether they work and are appropriate for the population.

While health promotion activities can be difficult to evaluate there are some excellent published examples of what works.

One example is the following umbrella review by Woldie *et al.* (2018). An umbrella review is a review of systematic reviews collecting all the available information on a topic to determine whether this is consistent, or if there are contradictory findings and if so, to explore why (Aromataris *et al.*, 2017).

The aim of this umbrella review was to examine evidence relating to the role of community health volunteers (CHVs) and how they contribute to improving access and use of essential health services in low- and middle-income countries (LMICs). In their final synthesis 39 qualitative and quantitative systematic reviews that both addressed the study aim and were of suitable methodological quality were included. These systematic reviews included a range of study designs.

The umbrella review was able to provide a typology of titles given to CHVs and the roles they undertook, which ranged from providing education to encouraging uptake of care, to supporting or facilitating behaviour change, to distributing drugs and providing counselling in their communities. The role that was most common was providing information and education about maternal and child health. CHVs worked with a range of diseases/health conditions including physical and mental conditions, communicable and non-communicable diseases and health promotion activities, such as immunisation services and adolescent health services. Some of the included reviews reported how CHVs were selected. Several of the reviews reported that when CHVs were involved in activities in primary healthcare settings this improved access and use by the community, which in turn improved population health outcomes.

Barriers and facilitators were also identified that impacted on CHV-led interventions, divided into community factors, health system factors and volunteer-related factors. Some of these are shown in *Table 11.2*.

**Table 11.2** *Barriers and facilitators impacting on CHV-led interventions*

| | |
|---|---|
| **Barriers** | ■ Community factors: limited ownership, disease-related stigma, gender roles and norms, lack of social recognition and acceptance, economic hardship and geographical difficulties<br>■ Health system factors: low or no payment/incentives, lack of supervision, limited training, lack of role definition, insufficient resources, lack of programme credibility, acceptability or appropriateness<br>■ Volunteer-related factors: inadequate space and time, limited access to community members, lack of knowledge of the community, poor follow-up, uncertainty on patient outcomes |
| **Facilitators** | ■ Community factors: respecting the volunteers, community participation and ownership, trust, involvement in selection and support of volunteers<br>■ Health system factors: provision of in-service training, supportive supervision and mentoring, recognition of role, integration into the formal health system<br>■ Volunteer-related factors: sense of altruism and social recognition, knowledge gain and career development, shared experience with the population served, feeling safe and secure |

(Woldie *et al.*, 2018, p. 1128)

The reviewers were able to articulate some key messages from the review that will support future CHV programmes:

- *Community health volunteers (CHVs) are lay individuals of varied background, coming from, or based in the communities they serve, who have received brief training on a health problem they have volunteered to engage with.*
- *It is evident that CHVs have the potential to supplement the formal health system in the struggle to achieve UHC [universal healthcare] in low- and middle-income countries (LMICs).*
- *Preventive, promotive and curative health services provided by CHVs were as good as, or in some cases better than those who are formally employed as health workers.*
- *In-service training, financial incentives, infrastructural support and supplies, appropriate monitoring, regular supportive supervision and evaluation, and integration of CHV programmes into the formal healthcare system were found to be facilitators of success.*

- Lack of regular supervision, limited training, lack of clear definition of roles, too many vertical programmes and insufficient resources were key barriers to success of volunteer-led health programmes.

(Woldie *et al.*, 2018. p. 1128)

You may recall that some of the discussions in *Chapter 8* resonate with these findings.

> **ACTIVITY 11.8**
>
> See if you can find a systematic review of a health promotion activity you are interested in.
>
> Make a list of the key messages and think how you could apply these to your activity.

## 11.6 Evidence-based health promotion in action

There are numerous examples in the literature where health promotion activities have either been tested in primary research studies using established research methods to investigate whether a health promotion activity works or not, or to see what people think about a health promotion activity, or secondary research where evidence has been synthesised to make recommendations for 'best practice' or 'future research'. In this section we will consider examples of primary and secondary research that have explored the effectiveness and suitability of health promotion activities in action.

### 11.6.1 Primary research study – a randomised controlled trial

The following is an example of a study which used a randomised controlled trial (considered 'gold standard' research for studies of effectiveness) to investigate whether a programme to help children manage weight was effective, through implementation of a programme called Families for Health, which included children and parents. The study was called: 'Randomised controlled trial evaluating the effectiveness and cost-effectiveness of "Families for Health", a family-based childhood obesity treatment intervention delivered in a community setting for ages 6 to 11 years' (Robertson *et al.*, 2017). The full study can be accessed at bit.ly/11-6-1.

A parenting approach called Families for Health was developed, which was aimed at helping parents to develop their skills in changing family lifestyles. The study was conducted at three sites in the UK and included children aged 6–11 years and their parents. This study was to evaluate Families for Health version 2 after Families for Health version 1 showed effective reductions in body mass index (BMI) in an initial smaller study (known as a pilot study) which included 27 children and their families.

Families for Health version 2 was run in the community. Participants were recruited to the trial through targeted methods (referral from a healthcare professional or a letter from the National Child Measurement programme), or through self-referral from people who had heard about the programme from adverts such as flyers and posters, or in the media.

> **ACTIVITY 11.9**
>
> Think about recruitment methods that you been involved in for health promotion interventions.
>
> Did people self-refer or were they referred by other health, social or educational professionals? Was there a difference between groups?

Families were eligible to take part if they had at least one child aged between 6–11 years who was overweight, the parents and children could speak English and the child did not have any medical reasons for being overweight or a behavioural problem that would limit them taking part in the study. A total of 115 families were recruited, including 128 children. From the recruited families, 56 families were randomised to the intervention (Families for Health version 2) and 59 families to a control group where they received usual care. Some families dropped out of both the intervention and control groups during the trial or were lost to follow-up.

> **ACTIVITY 11.10**
>
> Consider why people drop out of trials. Make a list of possible reasons.

The intervention group (Families for Health version 2) attended a family-based group programme with other families. This was run on a Saturday morning or afternoon for 10 weeks, each session lasting 2.5 hours. There were separate parents' and children's groups, although parents and children met mid-way through for a healthy snack and active game. The parents' programme consisted of parenting skills related to behaviour and relationships, healthy eating and physical activity. The children's programme focused on healthy eating, increasing physical activity and time to discuss their emotions. The course was run by specially trained facilitators.

The control group (usual care) was different in each of the three study areas. Those in Site A took part in a programme called 'One Body One Life' which was a group-based family intervention, Site B took part in 'Change4Life', a one-to-one support programme, which initially included a home visit but towards the end of the study changed to telephone counselling. Site C participants either attended a weight management programme, 'Weight Watchers' or were referred to the school nurse to be weighed and measured and receive advice. The care the control group received was therefore quite variable.

> **ACTIVITY 11.11**
>
> Consider: what are the difficulties researchers face when trying to compare groups where the participants in the intervention all receive the same care and the participants in the control group receive different types of care?

Follow-up was planned to take place at 3 and 12 months post-randomisation. However, some families had to wait to start Families for Health version 2 as there had to be a minimum of eight families before it was considered viable to run the programme, so the 3-month follow-up was therefore delayed. In some cases, the 3- and 12-month follow-up had to be combined, as families had waited so long to take part in the programme. For the control groups receiving usual care their 3-month visit took place regardless of whether they had accessed the usual care intervention.

To measure whether the study worked the authors used what is known as an anthropometric measure, which is a measurement of the proportions of the human body. The main or primary outcome measured was change in the children's BMI at 12 months compared with the control group; other outcomes measured were waist circumference, percentage body fat and parent weight and height (BMI). Changes in physical activity and diet were measured through an accelerometer that the children wore which measured movement, an activity diary that the children filled in with the help of their parents, a questionnaire about daily activity including fruit and vegetable consumption and a questionnaire about family eating and activity. The physical and mental health of children and their parents were measured using validated tools, as were family relationships and economic outcomes.

### ACTIVITY 11.12

Consider: what do we mean by a validated tool?
Make a list of validated tools you have seen used in health promotion activities.

The overall conclusion of the study was that the Families for Health version 2 programme was not clinically effective or cost-effective in managing weight in children, compared with usual care. There were no significant differences in physical activity, fruit and vegetable consumption or health-related quality of life between children in intervention and control groups. There were no differences in BMI at the 12-month follow-up between the children in the Families for Health group and those in the usual care group. The Families for Health intervention was delivered as planned, although some families had to wait to receive it. Overall the intervention was more expensive than usual care; parents' and children's experience was, however, positive.

### ACTIVITY 11.13

Read the study by Robertson *et al.* (2017) available at <u>bit.ly/11-6-1</u>.
- Why did the researchers think the Families for Health intervention did not work? Read p. 115 of the report and make some notes.
- What can you learn from this study about this type of intervention; what did the researchers suggest? Read p. 117 of the report and make some notes.
- Make a list of studies you have read where a health promotion intervention did or did not work. Which are most commonly reported: positive or negative results?

## 11.6.2 Evidence synthesis

An excellent example of an evidence synthesis was one undertaken by Flynn *et al.* (2005) which focused on reducing obesity and related chronic disease risk in children and youth. In this evidence synthesis the authors conducted a comprehensive search of all published literature including grey literature (information not produced by traditional publishers, such as conference presentations, theses, research reports, government reports, policy papers) and literature sourced from the internet.

The aim of this synthesis was to summarise what we know about health promotion programmes aimed at preventing and treating childhood obesity, to find out what works and to identify research gaps. The team who produced the review included research staff who spoke a variety of languages so were able to include papers written in French and Spanish as well as English, an expert advisory panel with a range of expertise, and collaborators from a variety of areas such as community development programmes, paediatric dietitians, immigration health and diverse urban community support facilitators.

Following the initial search, 147 studies were finally included in the synthesis, all of which had been subject to a rigorous appraisal process to ensure they were of sufficient quality to include. This review particularly highlights the difficulties of applying quality appraisal scoring systems designed for traditional research studies to health promotion studies. By their nature health promotion studies mirror real-life problems and as such, are often unable to be as thorough as tightly controlled trials that examine medical interventions, such as medication use, for example. Some of the studies had low recruitment or retention rates, some did not have comparison groups and others failed to take into account other issues that could have affected the study results, such as age, ethnicity, socioeconomic status and parental weight (these are known in research as confounding factors; things that influence the study outcomes other than the factor under investigation, e.g. the health promotion intervention).

The authors developed an approach where they appraised the studies from four perspectives:
- programme evaluation
- methodological rigour
- population health
- immigrant health.

They then used a system to score the studies, that was developed particularly for this type of review:
- Programme evaluation appraisal included assessing whether stakeholders had been involved in designing, implementing and evaluating the study, the ethics of the study and how useful and feasible it was over time.
- Methodological rigour was evaluated using validated appraisal tools.
- Population health appraisal considered whether programmes had included multidimensional approaches and healthy living strategies.

- Immigration health appraisal reviewed how studies had recruited participants and whether they had considered gender, religion and culture, food activity and customs.

The results were presented in three categories: a gap analysis, best practice in programme development and programme effectiveness. The gap analysis showed, for example, that there were limited programmes for the early life stage (0–5 years), there were few programmes that addressed gender-specific differences, only just over a quarter of programmes had follow-up periods of more than one year, no programmes specifically focused on immigrants and the most common interventions were diet, physical activity or both.

In terms of best practice in programme development, best practice was noted where stakeholder input was included at every step. Few studies considered the impact of the programme leader or facilitator, which can be a crucial indicator of programme performance. For programme effectiveness, knowledge was the least reported outcome. Most programmes in clinical and school settings showed improvement in body composition. Physical activity interventions showed good outcomes on body composition, nutrition, knowledge and chronic disease risk factors.

While this evidence synthesis was conducted 15 years ago, and results should be taken in context with more recent research, it is an excellent example of how the evidence underpinning health promotion interventions can be considered, appraised, synthesised and used to provide recommendations both for practice and future research. It also shows the difficulties that can be involved in determining which health promotion activities are more effective than others, as so many other factors can influence the results.

### ACTIVITY 11.14

Read the open access study by Flynn *et al.* (2005), available at bit.ly/A11-14, particularly the discussion, and consider why guidelines and task forces are often unable to make firm recommendations on health promotion interventions.

If you were designing a health promotion intervention, what recommendations do Flynn *et al.* (2005) suggest should be included?

### KEY LEARNING POINTS

Three key points to take away from *Chapter 11*:
- ☑ Evidence-based healthcare consists of evidence from research, professional expertise and patient preference, and should always take into account the context of the care delivery.
- ☑ Health promotion activities can be extremely complex and not always easy to evaluate; human and resource factors need to be considered when evaluating the effectiveness and appropriateness of health promotion activities.
- ☑ To ensure health promotion activities are both cost-effective and clinically effective, practitioners should always investigate the underpinning evidence before implementing activities.

# REFERENCES

Aromataris, E., Fernandez, R., Godfrey, C. et al. (2017) 'Umbrella reviews'. In Aromataris, E. and Munn, Z. (eds) *JBI Reviewer's Manual*. The Joanna Briggs Institute. Available at: https://reviewersmanual.joannabriggs.org/ (accessed 19 May 2020)

Cambridge Dictionary (2019a) *Evidence*. Cambridge University Press. Available at: https://dictionary.cambridge.org/dictionary/english/evidence (accessed 19 May 2020)

Cambridge Dictionary (2019b) *Evidence-based*. Cambridge University Press. Available at: https://dictionary.cambridge.org/dictionary/english/evidence-based (accessed 19 May 2020)

Donnelly, C., Boyd, I., Campbell, P. et al. (2018) Four principles to make evidence synthesis more useful for policy. *Nature*, **558:** 361–4. Available at: www.nature.com/articles/d41586-018-05414-4 (accessed 19 May 2020)

Evidence-Based Medicine Working Group (1992) Evidence-based medicine: a new approach to teaching the practice of medicine. *JAMA*, **268(17):** 2420–5.

Flynn, M., McNeil, D., Maloff, B. et al. (2005) Reducing obesity and related chronic disease risk in children and youth: a synthesis of evidence with 'best practice' recommendations. *Obesity Reviews*, **7(s1):** 7–66. Available at: https://onlinelibrary.wiley.com/doi/full/10.1111/j.1467-789X.2006.00242.x (accessed 19 May 2020)

Glasziou, P. (2011) Foreword. In Howick, J. *The Philosophy of Evidence-Based Medicine*. Wiley-Blackwell.

Hicks, N. (1997) *Evidence-based Health Care*. Available at: www.bandolier.org.uk/band39/b39-9.html (accessed 19 May 2020)

Lizarondo, L. and McArthur, A. (2017) Strategies for effective facilitation as a component of an evidence-based clinical fellowship program. *J Contin Educ Nurs*, **48(10):** 458–63.

Robertson, W., Fleming, J., Kama, I. et al. (2017) Randomised controlled trial evaluating the effectiveness and cost-effectiveness of 'Families for Health', a family-based childhood obesity treatment intervention delivered in a community setting for ages 6 to 11 years. *Health Technology Assessment*, **21(1)**. Available at: www.journalslibrary.nihr.ac.uk/hta/hta21010#/abstract (accessed 19 May 2020)

Rychetnik, L. and Wise, M. (2004) Advocating evidence-based health promotion: reflections and a way forward. *Health Promotion International*, **19(2):** 247–57. Available at: https://doi.org/10.1093/heapro/dah212 (accessed 19 May 2020)

Rycroft-Malone, J., McCormack, B., Hutchinson, A. et al. (2012) Realist synthesis: illustrating the method for implementation research. *Implementation Science*, **7:** 33. DOI:10.1186/1748-5908-7-33

What Works Network (2018) *The What Works Network: five years on*. Available from https://assets.publishing.service.gov.uk/government/uploads/system/uploads/attachment_data/file/677478/6.4154_What_works_report_Final.pdf (accessed 19 May 2020)

Woldie, M., Feyissa, G., Admasu, B. et al. (2018) Community health volunteers could help improve access to and use of essential health services by communities in LMICs: an umbrella review. *Health Policy and Planning*, **33(10):** 1128–43. DOI:10.1093/heapol/czy094

World Health Organization (2019) *Global Programme on Health Promotion Effectiveness (GPHPE)*. Available at: www.who.int/healthpromotion/areas/gphpe/en/ (accessed 19 May 2020)

# Index

Acheson report, 9, 48
Action on Smoking and Health (ASH), 10
Adverse Childhood Experiences (ACEs), 51
advocating, 12, 88–9, 95
alcohol, 9, 10, 22, 25, 26, 36, 51, 57, 58, 90, 91, 93, 94, 96, 106, 127, 129, 155, 173
Alzheimer's disease, 24–5, 76
artefact, 47
arthritis, 55, 76
assessing health needs, 107–11
asthma, 110
attitudes, 33, 34, 35, 41, 56, 95, 97
autism, 72, 113, 132

barriers, 27, 33–7, 53, 60, 61, 81, 97, 112, 113, 121, 126, 133, 144, 147, 190, 191
Beattie's model of health promotion, 29–31
behavioural change, 21–41
behavioural change wheel, 28, 37
beliefs, 5, 7, 8, 33, 34–6, 56, 93, 95, 112, 122, 128, 157, 158, 170
Beta Cell Education Resources for Training (BERTIE), 31–2
bioecological systems theory, 98–9
biomedical model of care, 127, 128, 158, 159, 161, 162
birth, 6, 59, 95
Black Report, 47, 50
Bradshaw's taxonomy of need, 107
BRCA1 gene, 76
BRCA2 gene, 76
breastfeeding, 14, 16

cancer, 5, 11, 32, 45, 46, 55, 57, 76, 79, 94, 96, 147, 173
cardiovascular disease, 25, 28, 46, 51, 55, 59, 76, 79, 96, 173

childhood and adolescence, 51, 90–4, 146, 173, 190
childhood mental health, 133
climate change, 7, 70
COM-B (Capacity Opportunity and Motivation = Behaviour) model, 35–6
communicable disease, see infectious diseases
community, 139–40, 228, 190
   and health, 140
   action, 61, 85, 142–64
Communities that Care system, 145
competence framework, 78
coronavirus, 71, 164
coronary heart disease, see cardiovascular disease
culture, 5, 49–50, 59, 97, 134, 179
cystic fibrosis, 76

Dahlgren and Whitehead's model, 22–3, 80–1, 103–4
decision-making, 31, 112, 158
dementia, 24, 25, 26, 55, 90, 96
depression, 57, 58, 96, 122, 128, 129, 141
deprivation, 46, 49, 53, 60–1, 145
determinants of health, 9, 22–5, 47–8, 52, 80–1, 96, 103–6
diabetes, 10, 30, 31–2, 40, 76, 96
diet, 9, 10, 14, 25, 26, 28, 34, 36, 47, 49, 51, 53, 60, 79, 90, 91, 94, 96, 125, 193, 195
   see also nutrition
disempowerment, 53–4
Dose Adjustment For Normal Eating (DAFNE), 31, 32

early years, 51, 91–2
Eatwell campaign, 27, 28, 29, 32
educational standards, 154–7, 159

197

# Index

emotional intelligence, 122, 124, 129, 171, 173
employment, 23, 46, 47, 48, 52–3, 54, 57, 62
empowerment, 29–30, 87, 111–12, 146
enabling, 86–7
engagement, 25, 27, 32, 142, 143, 146, 161
epidemiology, 71–3
equality and diversity, 97–8
ethical issues, 157–9
ethical principles, 158
    autonomy, 158, 159
    beneficence, 158
    justice, 158, 159, 189
    non-maleficence, 158
ethnicity, 59–62
evidence-based practice, 184–6
evidence synthesis, 187, 194–5
exercise, see physical activity
external locus of control, 112

fiscal change, 11, 14, 15
food advertising, 10
Food Standards Agency, 10
fragile X syndrome, 76
functional ability, 90

gambling, 11, 88, 89
gender, 55–9, 94–6
gender fluidity, 58–9
genetics, 73–8
genomics, 73–80
global health, 12, 69, 163–4
goal setting, 38–9, 117–18

hazards, 11, 52, 57, 60, 94, 95
HbA1c, 31, 39, 40
health (definition), 1–4
Health Act 2006, 105, 106, 142
health behaviours, 57, 94, 154
health belief model, 112–14
health education, 6–7, 27, 31–2
health impact assessments, 110–12
health improvement, 119, 140, 159
health literacy, 6, 111–12, 160–1
health needs analysis, 103
health needs assessment, 108–9
health promotion definition, 5–8
health protection, 12, 15, 27, 105
health screening, 79–80
Healthy Public Policy, 21, 85, 103, 105, 106

heart disease, see cardiovascular disease
holistic approach, 2, 3, 4, 5, 8, 12, 125, 130, 131, 179
Huntington's disease, 76
hypertension, see raised blood pressure

income, 48, 50, 51, 52, 53, 57, 61, 62, 90, 163
    categories, 163–4
inequalities in health, 9, 45–62, 95–6, 133–4, 144–5
infancy, 91
infectious diseases, 7, 8, 14, 60, 72, 164, 190
interagency working, 10
internal locus of control, 112

Johari window, 123, 172
joint strategic needs assessment, 109, 110

labelling, 128
large scale approaches, 26–8, 32
lay concepts of health, 4–5
leadership, 167–80
    compassionate leader, 179
    definition, 168–71
    health promotion, 179
    theories, 169
    transformational, 170
leading for change, 176–7
legislative change, 11, 15, 27, 30
LGBTQ (lesbian, gay, bisexual, transgender and queer/questioning), 58–9
life course, 51, 90–7
life expectancy, 45, 48, 49, 53, 94, 96, 130, 145
lifestyle, 9, 10, 22, 25, 26, 49, 60, 94, 96, 173, 191–3
living conditions, 8, 51, 60
loneliness, 96

Making Every Contact Count (MECC), 6, 26, 117, 129
Marfan syndrome, 76
Marmot Review, 9, 24, 48, 49, 50, 51, 52, 53, 54, 91, 95, 145
materialist model, 47, 50
measles, 112, 113, 117
mediating, 87–8
medical model, 2, 128, 162
men's health, 55–7, 94–5
mental activity, 25

mental health, 58, 121–34
    inequalities, 133–4
mental wellbeing, 51, 57, 91, 124, 125, 132
migrant health, 147
migration, 60–1
Millennium Development Goals, 13
MMR, *see* vaccination
mobility, 4, 145, 178
moral judgements, 158
morbidity, 46, 48, 49
mortality, 46, 48, 49, 94, 95
motivation, 28, 31, 34, 35, 36, 38, 81, 117, 143, 160
motivational interviewing, 38, 117
musculoskeletal conditions, 3, 4

neighbourhood, 60, 98, 140, 141, 142
    friendships, 145
NHS England, 10, 27, 88, 117
Nursing and Midwifery Council (NMC), 1, 2, 5, 7, 8, 52, 58, 122, 153–9, 162
nutrition, 8, 14, 15, 27, 28, 195
    *see also* diet
Nutrition Skills for Life, 27, 28

obesity, 10, 14, 15, 16, 27, 96, 194
    childhood, 10, 191, 194
older people, 96
organisational responsibilities, 97, 161
Ottawa Charter, 5, 6, 12, 13, 14, 85, 86, 105, 124

Pender's health promotion model, 35
person-centred approach, 2, 3, 4, 5, 7, 112, 117, 129
pharmacological interventions, 10, 162
physical activity, 9, 10, 15, 22, 25, 26, 51, 90, 96, 106, 155, 159, 192, 195
policy, 28, 30, 37, 47, 48, 81, 85, 103–11, 132, 157, 162–3, 178
pollution, 11, 60, 111, 106
positive working environment, 161
poverty, 50, 53, 57, 60, 62, 80, 133
preconception, 91
predisposing factors, 22, 25
pregnancy, 6, 91
prevention (primary, secondary and tertiary), 23, 25, 26, 28, 79

Prochaska and DiClemente's stages of change model, 39, 40, 115, 117
psychosis, 122
psychosocial model, 49, 50–1
public health, 8–12
Public Health Agency Northern Ireland, 24, 105, 132, 177
Public Health Scotland, 104, 177
Public Health Wales, 27, 51, 177

quality of health, 3

raised blood pressure, 51, 76
realistic synthesis, 186
Recovery Star, 130–1
resilience, 125, 132
Rights Commission, 125, 148
role modelling, 159, 161
Royal College of Nursing (RCN), 7–8, 11, 38, 93, 156, 157

safeguarding, 92–3, 156–7
sanitation, 8, 23, 80, 140
self-awareness, 122–4, 171–2, 173
self-efficacy, 112, 114, 115
self-esteem, 35, 51, 52, 112, 130
service user, 70, 110, 124, 177, 179
sexual health, 87, 94, 112
sickle cell anaemia, 45, 76, 79, 91
smoking, 9, 10, 22, 25, 26, 47, 49, 50, 94, 96, 173
    ban, 142
    cessation, 91, 93, 96, 112, 114, 115–16, 117, 155
social capital, 140–1, 143, 144
social change, 28, 62, 162
social determinants, 80, 81, 104, 105, 133
social engagement, 25
social gradient of health, 45–6
social inclusion, 22
social inequalities, 9, 47, 51
social media, 7, 88, 114, 125, 139
social need
    comparative, 107, 108, 109
    expressed, 107
    felt, 107
    normative, 107
social selection, 47
social support, 25, 50, 52, 133
socialisation, 51, 56

socioeconomic status, 91, 194
Soft Drinks Industrial Levy, 27
Spirit Level, 50
stages of change model, 28, 39–41, 115–16
stop smoking, *see* smoking cessation
stigma, 121, 123, 126, 127, 134, 190
stress, 26, 50, 51, 52, 60, 87, 125, 129, 130, 161, 176
SunSmart programme, 32
sustainable development goals, 14, 70, 94

Tannahill's model of health promotion, 26-7
theory of reasoned action, 33, 114
tobacco consumption, *see* smoking
transport, 81, 90, 106, 178

vaccination, 11, 72, 91, 92, 94, 96, 105, 112–14, 155, 159
values, 7, 111, 128, 144, 158, 162, 170, 171, 176, 179
voluntary sector, 111, 107, 164
vulnerable adults, 105, 106

Welsh Health Survey, 27
Whitehall study, 47
women's health, 55–7, 95–6
work, *see* employment
working conditions, 12, 52, 60